# Gastrointestinal Neoplasia

*Editors*

PAUL J. LIMBURG
DAN A. DIXON

# GASTROENTEROLOGY CLINICS OF NORTH AMERICA

www.gastro.theclinics.com

*Consulting Editor*
GARY W. FALK

September 2016 • Volume 45 • Number 3

**ELSEVIER**

1600 John F. Kennedy Boulevard • Suite 1800 • Philadelphia, Pennsylvania, 19103-2899
http://www.theclinics.com

GASTROENTEROLOGY CLINICS OF NORTH AMERICA Volume 45, Number 3
September 2016 ISSN 0889-8553, ISBN-13: 978-0-323-46257-0

Editor: Kerry Holland
Developmental Editor: Alison Swety

*Gastroenterology Clinics of North America* (ISSN 0889-8553) is published quarterly by Elsevier Inc., 360 Park Avenue South, New York, NY 10010-1710. Months of issue are March, June, September, and December. Business and Editorial Offices: 1600 John F. Kennedy Blvd., Suite 1800, Philadelphia, PA 19103-2899. Customer Service Office: 6277 Sea Harbor Drive, Orlando, FL 32887-4800. Periodicals postage paid at New York, NY and additional mailing offices. Subscription prices are $320.00 per year (US individuals), $100.00 per year (US students), $587.00 per year (US institutions), $350.00 per year (Canadian individuals), $720.00 per year (Canadian institutions), $445.00 per year (international individuals), $220.00 per year (international students), and $720.00 per year (international institutions). Foreign air speed delivery is included in all *Clinics* subscription prices. All prices are subject to change without notice. **POSTMASTER**: Send address changes to *Gastroenterology Clinics of North America*, Elsevier Health Sciences Division, Subscription Customer Service, 3251 Riverport Lane, Maryland Heights, MO 63043. **Telephone: 1-800-654-2452 (U.S. and Canada); 314-447-8871 (outside U.S. and Canada). Fax: 314-447-8029. E-mail: journalscustomerservice-usa@elsevier.com (for print support); journalsonlinesupport-usa@elsevier.com (for online support).**

*Reprints.* For copies of 100 or more, of articles in this publication, please contact the Commercial Reprints Department, Elsevier Inc., 360 Part Avenue South, New York, New York 10010-1710. Tel. 212-633-3874, Fax: 212-633-3820, E-mail: reprints@elsevier.com.

*Gastroenterology Clinics of North America* is also published in Italian by Il Pensiero Scientifico Editore, Rome, Italy; and in Portuguese by Interlivros Edicoes Ltda., Rua Commandante Coelho 1085, 21250 Cordovil, Rio de Janeiro, Brazil.

*Gastroenterology Clinics of North America* is covered in *MEDLINE/PubMed (Index Medicus)*, *Excerpta Medica*, *Current Contents/Clinical Medicine*, *Science Citation Index*, *ISI/BIOMED*, and *BIOSIS*.

# Contributors

## CONSULTING EDITOR

**GARY W. FALK, MD, MS**
Professor of Medicine, Division of Gastroenterology, Hospital of the University of Pennsylvania, University of Pennsylvania Perelman School of Medicine, Philadelphia, Pennsylvania

## EDITORS

**PAUL J. LIMBURG, MD, MPH, AGAF**
Professor of Medicine, Mayo Clinic College of Medicine, Rochester, Minnesota

**DAN A. DIXON, PhD**
Associate Professor of Cancer Biology, University of Kansas Medical Center, Kansas City, Kansas

## AUTHORS

**PAULINE AFCHAIN, MD**
Oncology Unit, Saint Antoine Hospital, APHP, Paris, France

**DAVID A. AHLQUIST, MD**
Carol M. Gatton Professor of Digestive Diseases Research Honoring Peter Carryer, MD, Division of Gastroenterology & Hepatology, Mayo Clinic, Rochester, Minnesota

**DENNIS J. AHNEN, MD, AGAF, FACG**
Professor of Medicine, University of Colorado School of Medicine, Aurora, Colorado

**BENJAMIN R. ALSOP, MD**
Clinical Assistant Professor, Department of Gastroenterology and Hepatology, Kansas City VA Medical Center, Kansas City, Missouri; Department of Gastroenterology and Hepatology, University of Kansas Medical Center, Kansas City, Kansas

**BRADLEY W. ANDERSON, MD**
Division of Gastroenterology & Hepatology, Mayo Clinic, Rochester, Minnesota

**THOMAS APARICIO, MD, PhD**
Gastroenterology and Digestive Oncology Unit, Avicenne Hospital, HUPSSD, APHP, Paris 13 University, Sorbonne Paris Cite, Bobigny, France

**RON BASUROY, MD, MBA**
Senior Research Fellow, Neuroendocrine Tumour Unit, Institute of Liver Studies, Kings College Hospital, Denmark Hill, London, United Kingdom

**LORI A. COBURN, MD**
Assistant Professor, Veterans Affairs Tennessee Valley Healthcare System and Division of Gastroenterology, Department of Medicine, Vanderbilt University School of Medicine, Nashville, Tennessee

**MARCIA CRUZ-CORREA, MD, PhD**
Professor, Departments of Medicine, Surgery and Biochemistry, University of Puerto Rico, Medical Sciences Campus, San Juan, Puerto Rico

**THOMAS RONALD JEFFRY EVANS, MB BS, MD, FRCP**
The Beatson West of Scotland Cancer Centre, University of Glasgow, Glasgow, United Kingdom

**MARÍA GONZÁLEZ-PONS, PhD**
Post Doctoral Fellow, University of Puerto Rico Comprehensive Cancer Center, San Juan, Puerto Rico

**ROBERT G. MAKI, MD, PhD, FACP**
Professor of Medicine, Tisch Cancer Institute, Mt Sinai Medical Center, New York, New York

**SYLVAIN MANFREDI, MD, PhD**
Hepato-Gastroenterology Unit, Dijon Hospital, Dijon, France

**JUAN M. MARQUÉS-LESPIER, MD**
Gastroenterology Fellow, Division of Gastroenterology, Department of Medicine, University of Puerto Rico School of Medicine, San Juan, Puerto Rico

**VIRGINIA MARTÍNEZ-MARÍN, MD, PhD**
Medical Oncology Service, Hospital Universitario La Paz, Madrid, Spain

**FLORENCE MARY, MD**
Gastroenterology and Digestive Oncology Unit, Avicenne Hospital, HUPSSD, APHP, Bobigny, France

**JOSHUA C. OBUCH, MD**
Fellow, Division of Gastroenterology & Hepatology, Department of Medicine, University of Colorado School of Medicine, Aurora, Colorado

**RICHARD M. PEEK Jr, MD**
Mina Cobb Wallace Professor, AGA Fellow, Division of Gastroenterology, Department of Medicine, Vanderbilt University School of Medicine, Nashville, Tennessee

**JOHN K. RAMAGE, MD, FRCP**
Professor, University of Winchester, Clinical Lead, Neuroendocrine Tumour Unit, Institute of Liver Studies, Kings College Hospital, Denmark Hill, London, United Kingdom

**PRATEEK SHARMA, MD**
Professor of Medicine, Department of Gastroenterology and Hepatology, Kansas City VA Medical Center, Kansas City, Missouri; Department of Gastroenterology and Hepatology, University of Kansas Medical Center, Kansas City, Kansas

**RAJ SRIRAJASKANTHAN, MD, FRCP**
Senior Lecturer and Consultant Physician, Neuroendocrine Tumour Unit, Institute of Liver Studies, Kings College Hospital, Denmark Hill, London, United Kingdom

**ELENA M. STOFFEL, MD, MPH**
Division of Gastroenterology, Department of Internal Medicine, University of Michigan Health System, Ann Arbor, Michigan

**JORDAN M. WINTER, MD**
Department of Surgery, Jefferson Pancreas, Biliary and Related Cancer Center, Thomas Jefferson University Hospital, Sidney Kimmel Medical College, Philadelphia, Pennsylvania

**LYDIA E. WROBLEWSKI, PhD**
Research Instructor, Division of Gastroenterology, Department of Medicine, Vanderbilt University School of Medicine, Nashville, Tennessee

**CINTHYA S. YABAR, MD**
Department of Surgery, Jefferson Pancreas, Biliary and Related Cancer Center, Thomas Jefferson University Hospital, Sidney Kimmel Medical College, Philadelphia, Pennsylvania

**AZIZ ZAANAN, MD, PhD**
Gastroenterology and Digestive Oncology Unit, Georges Pompidou Hospital, APHP, Paris Descartes University, Paris, France

# Contents

 Video content accompanies this article at http://www.gastro.
theclinics.com.

> Esophageal cancer carries a poor prognosis among gastrointestinal malignancies. Although esophageal squamous cell carcinoma predominates worldwide, Western nations have seen a marked rise in the incidence of esophageal adenocarcinoma that parallels the obesity epidemic. Efforts directed toward early detection have been difficult, given that dysplasia and early cancer are generally asymptomatic. However, significant advances have been made in the past 10 to 15 years that allow for endoscopic management and often cure in early stage esophageal malignancy. New diagnostic imaging technologies may provide a means by which cost-effective, early diagnosis of dysplasia allows for definitive therapy and ultimately improves the overall survival among patients.

> Gastric cancer (GC) is the third leading cause of cancer-related death. Only 28.3% of new GC cases survive more than 5 years. Although incidence has declined in the United States, an increase is estimated for 2016. Risk factors include sex (risk is higher in men), *Helicobacter pylori* infection, heredity, and lifestyle. GC is usually diagnosed between the ages of 60–80 years. Prognosis of GC is largely dependent on the tumor stage at diagnosis and classification as intestinal or diffuse type; diffuse-type GC has worse prognosis. Chemoprevention has been shown to decrease risk, but is currently not used clinically.

> Pancreatic cancer is now the third leading cause of cancer related deaths in the United States, yet advances in treatment options have been minimal over the past decade. In this article, we summarize the evaluation and treatments for this disease. We highlight molecular advances that hopefully will soon translate into improved outcomes.

> Small bowel adenocarcinomas (SBAs) are rare tumors, but their incidence is increasing. The most common primary location is the duodenum. Even

though SBAs are more often sporadic, some diseases are risk factors. Early diagnosis of small bowel adenocarcinoma remains difficult, despite significant radiologic and endoscopic progress. After R0 surgical resection, the main prognostic factor is lymph node invasion. An international randomized trial (BALLAD [Benefit of Adjuvant Chemotherapy For Small Bowel Adenocarcinoma] study) will evaluate the benefit of adjuvant chemotherapy. For metastatic disease, retrospectives studies suggest that platinum-based chemotherapy is the most effective treatment. Phase II studies are ongoing to evaluate targeted therapy in metastatic SBA.

Cancer is fundamentally a genetic disease caused by mutational or epigenetic alterations in DNA. There has been a remarkable expansion of the molecular understanding of colonic carcinogenesis in the last 30 years and that understanding is changing many aspects of colorectal cancer care. It is becoming increasingly clear that there are genetic subsets of colorectal cancer that have different risk factors, prognosis, and response to treatment. This article provides a general update on colorectal cancer and highlights the ways that genetics is changing clinical care.

The first 15 years of management of gastrointestinal stromal tumor (GIST) have led to 3 lines of therapy for metastatic disease: imatinib, sunitinib, and regorafenib. In the adjuvant setting, imatinib is usually given for 3 years postoperatively to patients with higher-risk primary tumors that are completely resected. In this review, issues regarding GIST adjuvant therapy are discussed. It is hoped this review will help the reader understand the present standard of care to improve upon it in years to come.

Neuroendocrine tumors are increasingly diagnosed, either incidentally as part of screening processes, or for symptoms, which have commonly been mistaken for other disorders initially. The diagnostic workup to characterize tumor behaviour and prognosis focuses on histologic, anatomic, and functional imaging assessments. Several therapeutic options exist for patients ranging from curative and debulking surgery through to liver-directed therapies and systemic treatments. Multimodal therapies are often required over the patient's disease history. The management paradigm can be complex but should be focused on curative resections and then on controlling symptoms and limiting disease progression. There are several new systemic therapies that have completed phase 3 studies with new compounds being studied in phase 2. Genetic and epigenetic markers may lead to a new era of personalised therapy in the future.

# GASTROENTEROLOGY CLINICS OF NORTH AMERICA

**THE CLINICS ARE AVAILABLE ONLINE!**
Access your subscription at:
www.theclinics.com

# Preface

# Gastrointestinal Neoplasia: Current Perspectives and Emerging Frontiers

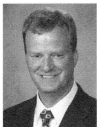 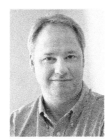

Paul J. Limburg, MD, MPH, AGAF          Dan A. Dixon, PhD
*Editors*

Gastrointestinal (GI) neoplasias present a substantial challenge to global public health, with recent data demonstrating that esophageal, gastric, colorectal, and pancreatic malignancies account for more than 3.1 million new and 2.1 million fatal cases per year.[1] In the United States, 2016 estimates indicate that incident cancers of the digestive system (304,930) will outnumber all other sites, including the genital system (297,530), respiratory system (243,820), and breast (249,260).[2] Encouragingly, favorable trends have been observed with respect to both incidence and mortality rates for many site-specific GI malignancies, although pancreas and small intestine cancers represent conspicuous exceptions.[3] To accelerate further progress, greater awareness and understanding are needed in the areas of molecular biology, epidemiology, early detection, diagnostic evaluation, clinical management, and survivorship, among others. In this issue of *Gastroenterology Clinics of North America*, these topics are reviewed by distinguished authors with expertise in neoplasia of the upper and lower GI tract, including GI stromal tumors and neuroendocrine tumors. State-of-the-science reviews for heritable syndromes, screening innovations, and role of the microbiome are also provided by leading authorities in these fields. Of note, hepatobiliary cancers are not addressed in this issue, to permit more thorough coverage of key concepts in luminal carcinogenesis.

We are indebted to the experts who so graciously contributed their time and talents to this important issue. By engaging a multidisciplinary, international team of collaborators, we strove to create an informative resource with broad application and appeal.

Gastroenterol Clin N Am 45 (2016) xi–xii
http://dx.doi.org/10.1016/j.gtc.2016.06.001
0889-8553/16/$ – see front matter © 2016 Published by Elsevier Inc.

**gastro.theclinics.com**

We appreciate your interest in the subject of GI neoplasia and hope that the content herein will be useful in your practice, research, and other professional endeavors.

Paul J. Limburg, MD, MPH, AGAF
Mayo Clinic College of Medicine
200 First Street SW
Rochester, MN 55905, USA

Dan A. Dixon, PhD
University of Kansas Medical Center
3901 Rainbow Boulevard
Kansas City, KS 66160, USA

E-mail addresses:
limburg.paul@mayo.edu (P.J. Limburg)
ddixon3@kumc.edu (D.A. Dixon)

## REFERENCES

1. Ferlay J, Soerjomataram I, Dikshit R, et al. Cancer incidence and mortality worldwide: sources, methods and major patterns in GLOBOCAN 2012. Int J Cancer 2015;136(5):E359–86.
2. Siegel RL, Miller KD, Jemal A. Cancer statistics, 2016. CA Cancer J Clin 2016; 66(1):7–30.
3. Howlader N, Noone AM, Krapcho M, et al. SEER Cancer Statistics Review. 1975–2012. Bethesda (MD): National Cancer Institute; 2015. Available at: http://seer.cancer.gov/csr/1975_2012/.

# Esophageal Cancer

 CrossMark

Benjamin R. Alsop, MD[a,b,]*, Prateek Sharma, MD[a,b]

## KEYWORDS

- Esophagus cancer • Esophageal squamous cell carcinoma
- Esophageal adenocarcinoma • Barrett's esophagus

## KEY POINTS

- Esophageal cancer is particularly deadly, with a 5-year survival in developed nations of 18%.
- Esophageal squamous cell carcinoma predominates in the developing world and worldwide, whereas esophageal adenocarcinoma (EAC) predominates in Western nations.
- Esophageal adenocarcinoma is commonly associated with GERD and obesity.
- Barrett's esophagus is a precursor of EAC; however, screening and surveillance remain controversial.

 Video content accompanies this article at http://www.gastro.theclinics.com.

## INTRODUCTION

Esophageal malignancy ranks sixth among cancer deaths worldwide.[1] It is estimated that just over 450,000 new cases of esophageal cancer were diagnosed in 2012, with around 400,000 deaths attributable to this condition in the same year.[2] Malignancies of the esophagus have a particularly poor prognosis because they typically cause no symptoms and thus are diagnosed late in their course. At this stage, resection and definitive cure are usually not an option. More than half present with distant metastases or unresectable disease.[3] This leads to a dismal 5-year survival that, although it has been increasing over time, remains a mere 18%.[4] There is a significant difference between developed and developing nations with respect to esophageal cancer incidence: it ranks 13th among all malignancies in the United States compared with 8th worldwide. Histology also differs, and although esophageal squamous cell carcinoma (ESCC) is more common throughout the world, esophageal adenocarcinoma (EAC) predominates in the United States.[2]

Disclosures: The authors have no relevant financial relationships to disclose.
a Department of Gastroenterology and Hepatology, Kansas City VA Medical Center, 4801 Linwood Boulevard, Kansas City, MO 64128, USA; b Department of Gastroenterology and Hepatology, University of Kansas Medical Center, 3901 Rainbow Boulevard, Mailstop 1023, Kansas City, KS 66160, USA
* Corresponding author. Department of Gastroenterology and Hepatology, Kansas City VA Medical Center, 4801 Linwood Boulevard, Kansas City, MO 64128.
E-mail address: benjamin.alsop@va.gov

Screening and surveillance for esophageal cancer have proven to be a difficult undertaking, given that esophageal symptoms (eg, gastroesophageal reflux disease [GERD]) correlate poorly with esophageal cancer and its precursor lesions. In fact, most patients diagnosed with early esophageal cancer lack any symptoms before the onset of dysphagia and weight loss that can signal an advanced-stage tumor. In cases where early esophageal cancer is detected, evolving therapies have not only improved the cure rate but have decreased the morbidity associated with treatment.

## SQUAMOUS CELL CARCINOMA OF THE ESOPHAGUS
### Demographics

Before 1990, ESCC was the predominant histologic subtype of esophageal cancer in the United States.[5] Since that time, however, there has been a decline of around 4% per year in the proportion of these cancers.[6] This is thought to be related to two main factors. First, the incidence of EAC is on the rise (see later). Second, there has been a steady decrease in the rates of tobacco and alcohol abuse, which are major contributors to ESCC, over that same time period. Although most ESCCs diagnosed in the United States are still found in white persons (including Hispanics), African Americans are disproportionately affected and account for 26% of cases.[6]

### Risk Factors

The risk factors for ESCC vary between developed and developing nations. In developing parts of the world, nutritional deficiencies and the subsequent lack of antioxidants that comes with a consistent diet of fruits and vegetables plays a role. Specifically, deficiencies in vitamins A, C, and E, and zinc, folate, and selenium contribute.[7] In industrialized countries, alcohol (>140 g/week) and tobacco use are known risk factors, with a synergistic effect in patients who abuse both.[8] Achalasia is associated with ESCC, likely caused by the effects of chronic stasis and inflammation in the esophagus. In fact, patients with achalasia are 28 times more likely to develop esophageal cancer than their unaffected counterparts. Despite this fact, given the low absolute risk, screening/surveillance strategies have failed to demonstrate a survival benefit and are not routinely recommended in these patients.[9]

Caustic ingestion, usually accidental in children and intentional in adolescents and adults, has been linked to ESCC. The incidence has been reported as somewhere between 2% and 30%, with an occurrence rate 1000 times that of age-matched individuals.[10] As with achalasia, the pathophysiology seems to be related to the chronic inflammation/regeneration of the squamous mucosa of the esophagus. In most patients, the development of dysplasia occurs over several decades; however, ESCC can develop in those whose ingestion occurred as recently as 1 year prior.[11]

Tylosis is an autosomal-dominant inherited condition known to predispose to ESCC, with patients typically also demonstrating hyperkeratosis of the hands and feet. This susceptibility is traced to a gene mutation on 17q25.1 that encodes for a protein central to EGFR signaling. In the presence of this mutation, affected patients have between 50% and 100% chance of development of ESCC.[12,13] The American Society for Gastrointestinal Endoscopy recommends screening endoscopy every 1 to 3 years in individuals with the identified mutation.[14]

## ADENOCARCINOMA OF THE ESOPHAGUS
### Demographics

EAC is on the rise in the Western world. A recent analysis of the trends in esophageal cancer diagnosis from the Surveillance, Epidemiology, and End Results database[5] demonstrated that over the past 30 years, the proportion of patients with EAC nearly doubled, from 35% to 61%. This change is attributed not only to the declining incidence of ESCC noted previously, but also the rise in obesity and related conditions over the same time period.

### Risk Factors

There is a clear link between GERD and EAC, and chronic exposure of the distal esophagus to acid is thought to be a critical aspect of the pathophysiology of this malignant transformation. It is thought that through the process of healing erosive esophagitis, metaplasia occurs and leads to formation of a premalignant columnar lining of the esophagus.[15] As a result, conditions that increase esophageal acid exposure are risk factors for EAC. Obesity, in particular, has been thought to contribute to the rising incidence of EAC in developed nations. Beyond the mechanical implications of the obese body habitus (eg, formation of hiatal hernia) and the net effect of increased acid exposure in the distal esophagus,[16] there is increasing evidence to suggest a link between the rise in serum adipokines in obese patients and the risk of EAC.[17] Finally, cigarette smoking is a risk factor for EAC, just as it is in many cancers.[7] Unlike ESCC, however, the link between EAC and alcohol use is not well-established.[18]

## BARRETT'S ESOPHAGUS

Although the presence of columnar-lined epithelium in the distal esophagus was first described in 1906 by Tileston,[19] it was Barrett's[20] subsequent article that led to the eponymous term "Barrett's esophagus." Barrett's esophagus is defined as a change in the normally squamous epithelium of the distal esophagus to a columnar type.[21] This gives the classic endoscopic appearance of salmon-colored mucosa, which also demonstrates the presence of goblet cells when examined under the microscope (**Fig. 1**A). This specialized intestinal metaplasia, or nondysplastic Barrett's esophagus, is thought to occur as a response to chronic inflammation and has an increased risk of further development into EAC. Patients diagnosed with Barrett's esophagus are more than 11 times more likely to develop esophageal cancer when compared with those without. This represents a yearly incidence of EAC between 0.12% and 0.36% in those affected.[22,23] Furthermore, the length of a Barrett's segment correlates positively with the risk of progression to high-grade dysplasia and EAC.[24] It should be noted, however, that although the relative risk of esophageal cancer is high in these patients, the absolute risk remains low; Barrett's esophagus can be found in 5% to 6% of the US population.[25]

Screening for Barrett's esophagus is a controversial undertaking. One particular difficulty with a screening program for esophageal malignancy is the selection of individuals who should undergo endoscopy. Based on its decreased relative prevalence when compared with colon cancer (4.4 vs 43.7/100,000[4]), for example, a population-wide screening effort similar to colonoscopy would be cost-prohibitive. Furthermore, Barrett's esophagus itself is an asymptomatic condition; most patients have chronic GERD symptoms reflective of the underlying disorder. Among all patients with GERD, only 5% to 15% are found to have Barrett's esophagus.[26] However, screening and surveillance continue to be recommended by various gastrointestinal societies in patients with multiple risk factors for EAC.[14,27,28]

On identification of Barrett's esophagus, patients are usually enrolled in a surveillance protocol. In patients with nondysplastic Barrett's esophagus, it is generally

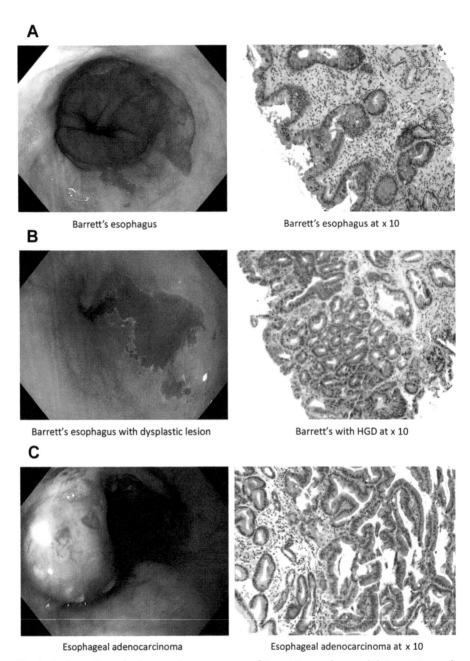

**Fig. 1.** Endoscopic and microscopic appearance of Barrett's esophagus. (*A*) Barrett's esophagus. (*B*) Barrett's esophagus with dysplastic lesion. (*C*) Esophageal adenocarcinoma. (*A–C*, H&E stain, original magnification ×10). (*Courtesy of* Rachel Cherian, MD, Kansas City, MO.)

accepted that surveillance esophagogastroduodenoscopy in these patients should be performed every 3 to 5 years,[28] with methodical documentation of the Barrett's extent[29] and standardized sampling[30] of the affected areas. This continues as long as there is no evidence of dysplastic progression.

A diagnosis of low-grade dysplasia carries a risk of progression between 0.3% and 0.8% per year.[31] It also poses a unique challenge because of only slight interobserver agreement in its characterization among pathologists (kappa = 0.14; overall 55.6%).[32] This is reflected in the guidelines for management of low-grade dysplasia in the setting of Barrett's esophagus. It is first recommended that two expert pathologists confirm the diagnosis. Once confirmed, it should be followed with endoscopy every 6 months for the first year, then yearly thereafter unless there is development of further dysplastic progression.

When a high-grade dysplastic lesion is identified within a Barrett's segment (**Fig. 1**B), the endoscopist and patient must decide whether to remove the lesion (endoscopic mucosal resection [EMR]) or pursue surgical resection. The risk of progression to adenocarcinoma in the setting of high-grade dysplasia is 6% per year.[33] It is recommended that any nodules found within a segment of Barrett's mucosa be removed, typically via EMR, because this allows for histologic evaluation and definitive staging of the lesion. After resection of the dysplastic segment, the remaining metaplastic epithelium should be removed until the distal esophagus once again is covered entirely by squamous (now termed neosquamous) epithelium (see the section on treatment). Surveillance endoscopy then continues, with systematic biopsies obtained over the extent of the previously columnar mucosa. Although rare, there have been reports of "buried" dysplasia and adenocarcinoma beneath the neosquamous epithelium following ablation of a Barrett's segment.[34]

## DIAGNOSIS

The diagnosis of esophageal cancer is most often preceded by symptoms of progressive dysphagia and, in many cases, weight loss. Chest pain occurs less often but may signal invasion of tumor into the mediastinum. Odynophagia may be present if there is significant ulceration of an esophageal lesion or severe esophagitis proximal to the obstruction. Asymptomatic patients may present with more insidious findings, such as anemia, mediastinal lymphadenopathy, or even hoarseness caused by recurrent laryngeal nerve encasement.

Occasionally, patients are first evaluated with a barium esophagram; this study would demonstrate narrowing of the lumen and dilation proximal to the level of the tumor. The gold standard for evaluation of worrisome esophageal symptoms is upper endoscopy, which allows not only visualization of a tumor but also tissue sampling for pathologic confirmation. Esophageal malignancy can present as a flat, subtle area or a lumen-obscuring mass (**Fig. 1**C). Persistent ulceration and refractory strictures of the esophagus should raise suspicion for malignancy. Given the wide range of presentations of this malignancy, the endoscopist must carefully evaluate the entire esophagus during an upper endoscopy. Because of implications for treatment (surgical planning, the need for stent placement, and posttreatment evaluation), it is imperative that the size, morphology, and proximal and distal extent of the tumor are carefully described in the endoscopy report. It is generally recommended that at least 7 biopsies be obtained to ensure adequacy of sample.[35] Brushings alone are inadequate, but if added to biopsy samples this brings the sensitivity to near 100%.

## STAGING

Staging of esophageal cancer is described using the American Joint Committee on Cancer's TNM system (**Table 1**).[36] This method allows for a description of the degree of tumor invasion (T), the number of regional lymph nodes involved (N), and any distant metastases (M). There is a clinically significant division between esophageal tumors

**Table 1**
**TNM (American Joint Committee on Cancer) staging of esophageal cancer**

**Esophageal Adenocarcinoma Clinical Staging**

| Stage | T | N | M | Grade |
|---|---|---|---|---|
| 0 | Tis (high-grade dysplasia) | N0 | M0 | 1, X |
| IA | T1 | N0 | M0 | 1–2, X |
| IB | T1 | N0 | M0 | 3 |
| | T2 | N0 | M0 | 1–2, X |
| IIA | T2 | N0 | M0 | 3 |
| IIB | T3 | N0 | M0 | Any |
| | T1–2 | N1 | M0 | Any |
| IIIA | T1–2 | N2 | M0 | Any |
| | T3 | N1 | M0 | Any |
| | T4a | N0 | M0 | Any |
| IIIB | T3 | N2 | M0 | Any |
| IIIC | T4a | N1–2 | M0 | Any |
| | T4b | Any | M0 | Any |
| | Any | N3 | M0 | Any |
| IV | Any | Any | M1 | Any |

**Esophageal Squamous Cell Carcinoma Clinical Staging**

| Stage | T | N | M | Grade | Tumor Location |
|---|---|---|---|---|---|
| 0 | Tis (high-grade dysplasia) | N0 | M0 | 1, X | Any |
| IA | T1 | N0 | M0 | 1, X | Any |
| IB | T1 | N0 | M0 | 2–3 | Any |
| | T2–3 | N0 | M0 | 1, X | Lower, X |
| IIA | T2–3 | N0 | M0 | 1, X | Upper, middle |
| | T2–3 | N0 | M0 | 2–3 | Lower, X |
| IIB | T2–3 | N0 | M0 | 2–3 | Upper, middle |
| | T1–2 | N1 | M0 | Any | Any |
| IIIA | T1–2 | N2 | M0 | Any | Any |
| | T3 | N1 | M0 | Any | Any |
| | T4a | N0 | M0 | Any | Any |
| IIIB | T3 | N2 | M0 | Any | Any |
| IIIC | T4a | N1–2 | M0 | Any | Any |
| | T4b | Any | M0 | Any | Any |
| | Any | N3 | M0 | Any | Any |
| IV | Any | Any | M1 | Any | Any |

*Abbreviations:* G, histologic grade; G1, well differentiated; G2, moderately differentiated; G3, poorly differentiated; G4, undifferentiated—stage grouping as G3 squamous; GX, grade cannot be assessed—stage grouping as G1; M, distant metastasis; M0, no distant metastasis; MI, distant metastasis; N, Regional lymph nodes; N0, no regional lymph node metastasis; N1, metastasis in 1–2 regional lymph nodes; N2, metastasis in 3–6 regional lymph nodes; N3, metastasis in 7 or more regional lymph nodes; NX, regional lymph nodes cannot be assessed; T, primary tumor; T0, no evidence of primary tumor; T1, tumor invades lamina propria, muscularis mucosae, or submucosa; T2, tumor invades muscularis propria; T3, tumor invades adventitia; T4, tumor invades adjacent structures; T1a, tumor invades lamina propria or muscularis mucosae; T1b, tumor invades submucosa; T4a, resectable tumor invading pleura, pericardium, or diaphragm. Unresectable tumor invading other; T4b, adjacent structures, such as the aorta, vertebral body, and trachea; Tis, high-grade dysplasia; Tx, primary tumor cannot be assessed.

Used with permission of the American Joint Committee on Cancer (AJCC), Chicago, Illinois. The original and primary source for this information is the AJCC Cancer Staging Manual, Seventh Edition (2010) published by Springer Science+Business Media.

that involve the submucosa (T1b) and beyond, from those that are limited to the mucosal layer (T1a, T0). **Fig. 2** demonstrates the principles of T-staging for tumors of the esophagus.

In patients with high-grade dysplasia/carcinoma-in-situ (T0) or intramucosal carcinoma (T1a), the risk of local lymph node involvement is low. It has been shown that patients with T0 tumors have essentially 0% chance of lymph node metastasis; in those with T1a lesions, the risk is only 1% to 2%.[37] Furthermore, there is also limited evidence that endoscopic resection of T1b lesions with only superficial involvement of the submucosa (sm1) is effective,[38] but this only applies to EAC. In such lesions, the diagnosis and therapy are achieved via resection of the mucosal layer. T1b ESCC prompts more aggressive therapy, with esophagectomy. Unfortunately, only about one in four EACs diagnosed in the United States today is of an early stage and amenable to endoscopic therapy,[39,40] and these are usually found during screening examinations rather than on investigation of symptoms.[21] However, the number of esophageal cancers being diagnosed at an early stage is increasing.[5]

When an invasive tumor is identified, staging is performed with a combination of several modalities. The process typically begins with computed tomography (CT) of the chest, abdomen, and pelvis using intravenous contrast to evaluate for any obvious lymphadenopathy or distal metastases. Another option is to perform hybrid PET/CT, which has a slightly higher yield than CT or PET alone and has demonstrated the ability to identify otherwise occult metastases.[41] This is important in avoiding unnecessary/ineffective surgical intervention in such patients. The most common sites of metastasis seen in esophageal cancer depend on tumor histology; ESCC spreads within the thorax, whereas EAC tends to spread within the abdomen and can be seen in the liver and peritoneum. The thoracoabdominal skeleton and adrenal glands can also be affected. When no obvious distant metastases are identified, locoregional staging is warranted. This is best performed with endoscopic ultrasound, which allows for better assessment of tumor invasion and regional lymph node involvement when

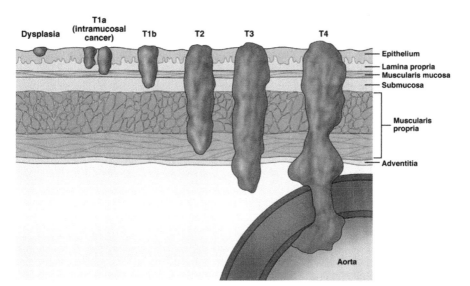

**Fig. 2.** Tumor staging of esophageal cancer. (*From* Rubenstein JH, Shaheen NJ. Epidemiology, diagnosis, and management of esophageal adenocarcinoma. Gastroenterology 2015;149(2):307; with permission.)

compared with CT, PET, or a combination of the two.[42] An added benefit of this modality is the ability to perform fine-needle aspiration of any suspicious lymph nodes during the procedure. It should be noted that although endoscopic ultrasound is the most accurate modality for establishing the T stage of a lesion, none of the imaging modalities discussed previously are adequate for this purpose in early lesions and occasionally overestimate their depth. For that reason, EMR should be the first step for evaluation of subtle/flat lesions.[43]

## TREATMENT

As with other malignancies, the treatment of esophageal cancer is directed by the stage. For intramucosal tumors (T0-T1a), endoscopic resection is diagnostic and curative. Most such early stage tumors are identified as part of an endoscopic screening/surveillance program in the setting of Barrett's esophagus. Techniques for resection of these lesions include EMR and endoscopic submucosal dissection (ESD). EMR involves cap-assisted resection with or without band ligation of the involved segment of the esophagus and is generally a piecemeal technique (see Video 1 for demonstration). It is much more widely available, because ESD requires significant additional training and expertise; at this time, only a few quaternary referral centers in the United States employ endoscopists with the adequate background and case volume to routinely perform such procedures. Long-term follow-up of 1000 patients with early EAC treated with EMR in one study demonstrated an impressive rate for complete remission (96.3%) and long-term complete remission (93.8%) rates, suggesting this is an effective and durable therapy.[44] Significant bleeding (1.4%), stricture formation (1.3%), and perforation (0.1%) were the only observed side effects of this therapy, all of which were managed endoscopically. In contrast to EMR, the major advantage to ESD is the ability to remove a lesion en bloc.[45] This is particularly important in the management of large, laterally spreading squamous cell carcinomas. The procedure uses submucosal injection of fluid to raise an esophageal lesion, followed by submucosal dissection underneath with grasping-type scissor knives and/or a needle-knife. Although not widely available yet in the United States, this technique has been shown to be safe and effective in high- and low-volume centers in Japan. The major complication, stricture formation, tends to occur only in cases where the resected specimen involves more than half the circumference of the esophagus.[46]

On resection of the tumor, it is then imperative that the remaining metaplastic epithelium is eradicated. The most commonly used method to accomplish this is radiofrequency ablation, which uses radiofrequency energy delivered via a catheter to the mucosa. Small, scope tip-affixed catheters allow for segmental ablation of metaplastic tissue under direct visualization; alternatively, 360-degree catheters allow for ablation of larger areas within the esophagus (see Video 1 for demonstration). With repeated applications of this technique, 80% to 90% of patients with dysplastic Barrett's experience complete eradication of intestinal metaplasia.[47] Postablation surveillance is critical, however, because up to 20% of patients experience a recurrence of Barrett's esophagus.[48] Cryotherapy and photodynamic therapy have also been used for this purpose.

The role of surgical therapy for early esophageal cancer (T0-T1b, sm1) continues to be debated. Although esophagectomy was the traditional approach to esophageal dysplasia in the past, management has gradually trended toward the less invasive endoscopic methods described previously. Surgical morbidity, when compared with an outpatient procedure, is one obvious drawback. A study of patients treated in two high-volume centers in Germany found a surgical complication rate of 32%, compared with 0% for endoscopic therapy.[49] However, the definitive nature of esophagectomy has to be weighed against the risk not only of recurrence in the endoscopic approach but the need for continued surveillance endoscopies. In the same study, the endoscopically treated cohort experienced a recurrence rate of cancer of 6.6%; all patients were retreated successfully.

For tumors that involve the deeper layers of the esophagus (T2 and beyond) and/or with nodal involvement, neoadjuvant therapy is recommended.[50] Either neoadjuvant (presurgical) chemotherapy[51] (typically a platinum-based regimen) or the combination of neoadjuvant chemotherapy and radiation[52] confers a survival benefit in such patients over surgical therapy alone. Furthermore, a combination of chemotherapy and radiation (chemoradiotherapy) is more efficacious than either of these two modalities alone.[53] The major mechanism by which chemotherapy and radiation work in synergy is through magnification of radiation damage via incorporation of the chemotherapy drug into DNA/RNA, followed by inhibition of the DNA repair process after radiation.[54]

When distant metastases have been identified, treatment options are severely limited and the focus shifts toward palliation. Median survival can be only 9 to 10 months despite treatment with chemotherapy.[55] It should be noted, however, that the choice of which patients to treat is critical; such factors as age, performance status, the presence of liver or peritoneal metastases, and serum chemistry values all influence response to chemotherapy.[56] One palliative measure that may not only help to facilitate nutrition but also allow for the comfort of continued oral intake is esophageal stent placement. Self-expandable metal stents that are either fully or partially covered with a synthetic membrane are placed endoscopically, with or without fluoroscopic guidance. Up to 90% of patients with esophageal cancer may see an improvement in dysphagia symptoms with the placement of an esophageal stent.[57] The main risk with esophageal stenting is migration into the stomach, which may require endoscopic retrieval. This is a particular concern in patients who undergo stent placement followed by chemotherapy that might shrink the tumor, thus allowing the stent to be displaced. Ultimately, enteral feeding may be accomplished through the use of a percutaneous endoscopic gastrostomy tube or radiologically placed gastrostomy tube in those patients who are either not candidates for esophageal stent placement or have failed this modality because of tumor ingrowth. Additionally, percutaneous endoscopic gastrostomy tubes are frequently placed for patients in anticipation of radiation therapy because of the odynophagia that often accompanies this treatment.

## THE FUTURE OF DIAGNOSIS AND MANAGEMENT

Although risk factor modification is a cornerstone of prevention, future research with the goal of further decreasing the incidence of esophageal cancer will undoubtedly be directed toward earlier detection. Perhaps the first step will be to better direct the resources of screening endoscopy toward those who need it most. This would involve more accurate predictive models based on known risk factors, genetic predisposition, and possibly even biomarkers for early disease and disease progression. For those with traditional risk factors who are referred for endoscopic evaluation, techniques have been developed with an increased sensitivity and specificity for dysplasia. Wide-area transepithelial sampling involves passing a brush over the mucosa of the Barrett's segment and submitting a block of cells for computer-assisted analysis. Early in vivo evaluations of this technology have demonstrated marked improvements in detection of metaplasia and dysplasia and interobserver variability among pathologists.[58,59] In an attempt to avoid the extensive tissue sampling and subsequent pathology costs of current surveillance protocols, advanced imaging modalities have been evaluated. The use of narrow-band imaging allows for differentiation of mucosal and vascular patterns along the surface of the esophageal mucosa; criteria have been established that can reliably predict the presence of dysplasia, thereby allowing for a more targeted biopsy approach.[60,61] Real-time pathology has been assessed through the use of volumetric laser endomicroscopy and probe-based confocal laser endomicroscopy, both of which would theoretically allow the endoscopist to diagnose and treat esophageal dysplasia in the same procedure.[62,63] It is hoped that future trials and expanding availability of these modalities will continue to improve not only the detection but also the outcomes in patients with early stage esophageal malignancy.

## OTHER ESOPHAGEAL MALIGNANCIES

Squamous cell carcinoma and adenocarcinoma make up most esophageal malignancies worldwide, but a few other rare types should be mentioned. Epithelial tumors include small cell carcinoma and melanoma, and verrucous carcinoma and carcinosarcoma, both of which are variants of ESCC. Lymphoma (secondary and less commonly primary) and gastrointestinal stromal cell tumors make up the nonepithelial malignancies of the esophagus. A detailed discussion of the characteristics of these rare tumors and their management is beyond the scope of this review.

## SUMMARY

Esophageal cancer is a malignancy with a poor 5-year survival. Nearly 500,000 people are diagnosed per year, worldwide. ESCC remains the prevalent histologic subtype of esophageal cancer around the globe, but Western nations have seen a predominance and rising incidence of EAC. Screening efforts for esophageal cancer have been thwarted by a poor correlation between symptoms and endoscopic findings, and most cancers are diagnosed at a late clinical stage. However, improvements in minimally invasive endoscopic therapy and radiation and systemic chemotherapy have provided some small benefits to survival and quality of life in these patients. Future research should be directed toward risk stratification, cost-effective care, and early detection of esophageal dysplasia and malignancy in the hope that measureable improvements can be made in the prognosis of those affected by this deadly cancer.

## SUPPLEMENTARY DATA

Supplementary data related to this article can be found at http://dx.doi.org/10.1016/j.gtc.2016.04.001.

## REFERENCES

1. Global Burden of Disease Cancer Collaboration, Fitzmaurice C, Dicker D, et al. The Global Burden of Cancer 2013. JAMA Oncology 2015;1(4):505–27.
2. Arnold M, Soerjomataram I, Ferlay J, et al. Global incidence of oesophageal cancer by histological subtype in 2012. Gut 2015;64(3):381–7.
3. Enzinger PC, Mayer RJ. Esophageal cancer. N Engl J Med 2003;349(23): 2241–52.
4. Peery AF, Crockett SD, Barritt AS, et al. Burden of Gastrointestinal, Liver, and Pancreatic Diseases in the United States. Gastroenterology 2015;149(7): 1731–41.e3.

5.  Njei B, McCarty TR, Birk JW. Trends in esophageal cancer survival in United States adults from 1973 to 2009: a SEER database analysis. J Gastroenterol Hepatol 2016. http://dx.doi.org/10.1111/jgh.13289.

6.  Trivers KF, Sabatino SA, Stewart SL. Trends in esophageal cancer incidence by histology, United States, 1998–2003. Int J Cancer 2008;123(6):1422–8.

7.  Engel LS, Chow WH, Vaughan TL, et al. Population attributable risks of esophageal and gastric cancers. J Natl Cancer Inst 2003;95(18):1404–13.

8.  Prabhu A, Obi KO, Rubenstein JH. The synergistic effects of alcohol and tobacco consumption on the risk of esophageal squamous cell carcinoma: a meta-analysis. Am J Gastroenterol 2014;109(6):822–7.

9.  Leeuwenburgh I, Scholten P, Alderliesten J, et al. Long-term esophageal cancer risk in patients with primary achalasia: a prospective study. Am J Gastroenterol 2010;105(10):2144–9.

10. Kay M, Wyllie R. Caustic ingestions in children. Curr Opin Pediatr 2009;21(5): 651–4.

11. Jain R, Gupta S, Pasricha N, et al. ESCC with metastasis in the young age of caustic ingestion of shortest duration. J Gastrointest Cancer 2010;41(2):93–5.

12. Stevens HP, Kelsell DP, Bryant SP, et al. Linkage of an American pedigree with palmoplantar keratoderma and malignancy (palmoplantar ectodermal dysplasia type III) to 17q24. Literature survey and proposed updated classification of the keratodermas. Arch Dermatol 1996;132(6):640–51.

13. Ellis A, Field JK, Field EA, et al. Tylosis associated with carcinoma of the oesophagus and oral leukoplakia in a large Liverpool family–a review of six generations. Eur J Cancer B Oral Oncol 1994;30B(2):102–12.

14. Evans JA, Early DS, Fukami N, et al. The role of endoscopy in Barrett's esophagus and other premalignant conditions of the esophagus. Gastrointest Endosc 2012; 76(6):1087–94.

15. Souza RF, Krishnan K, Spechler SJ. Acid, bile, and CDX: the ABCs of making Barrett's metaplasia. Am J Physiol Gastrointest Liver Physiol 2008;295(2):G211–8.

16. El-Serag HB, Ergun GA, Pandolfino J, et al. Obesity increases oesophageal acid exposure. Gut 2007;56(6):749–55.

17. Ryan AM, Healy LA, Power DG, et al. Barrett esophagus: prevalence of central adiposity, metabolic syndrome, and a proinflammatory state. Ann Surg 2008; 247(6):909–15.

18. Wu AH, Wan P, Bernstein L. A multiethnic population-based study of smoking, alcohol and body size and risk of adenocarcinomas of the stomach and esophagus (United States). Cancer Causes Control 2001;12(8):721–32.

19. Tileston W. Peptic ulcer of the oesophagus. Am J Med Sci 1906;132(2):240–65.

20. Barrett NR. Chronic peptic ulcer of the oesophagus and 'oesophagitis'. Br J Surg 1950;38(150):175–82.

21. Spechler SJ, Sharma P, Souza RF, et al. American Gastroenterological Association technical review on the management of Barrett's esophagus. Gastroenterology 2011;140(3):e18–52 [quiz: e13].

22. Hvid-Jensen F, Pedersen L, Drewes AM, et al. Incidence of adenocarcinoma among patients with Barrett's esophagus. N Engl J Med 2011;365(15):1375–83.

23. Kroep S, Lansdorp-Vogelaar I, Rubenstein JH, et al. An accurate cancer incidence in Barrett's esophagus: a best estimate using published data and modeling. Gastroenterology 2015;149(3):577–85.e4 [quiz: e14–5].

24. Anaparthy R, Gaddam S, Kanakadandi V, et al. Association between length of Barrett's esophagus and risk of high-grade dysplasia or adenocarcinoma in patients without dysplasia. Clin Gastroenterol Hepatol 2013;11(11):1430–6.

25. Hayeck TJ, Kong CY, Spechler SJ, et al. The prevalence of Barrett's esophagus in the US: estimates from a simulation model confirmed by SEER data. Dis Esophagus 2010;23(6):451–7.

26. Westhoff B, Brotze S, Weston A, et al. The frequency of Barrett's esophagus in high-risk patients with chronic GERD. Gastrointest Endosc 2005;61(2):226–31.

27. Spechler SJ, Sharma P, Souza RF, et al. American Gastroenterological Association medical position statement on the management of Barrett's esophagus. Gastroenterology 2011;140(3):1084–91.

28. Shaheen NJ, Falk GW, Iyer PG, et al. ACG clinical guideline: diagnosis and management of Barrett/'s esophagus. Am J Gastroenterol 2016;111(1):30–50.

29. Sharma P, Dent J, Armstrong D, et al. The development and validation of an endoscopic grading system for Barrett's esophagus: the Prague C & M criteria. Gastroenterology 2006;131(5):1392–9.

30. Reid BJ, Blount PL, Feng Z, et al. Optimizing endoscopic biopsy detection of early cancers in Barrett's high-grade dysplasia. Am J Gastroenterol 2000; 95(11):3089–96.

31. Singh S, Manickam P, Amin AV, et al. Incidence of esophageal adenocarcinoma in Barrett's esophagus with low-grade dysplasia: a systematic review and meta-analysis. Gastrointest Endosc 2014;79(6):897–909.e1 [quiz: 983.e1, 983.e3].

32. Wani S, Falk GW, Post J, et al. Risk factors for progression of low-grade dysplasia in patients with Barrett's esophagus. Gastroenterology 2011;141(4):1179–86, 1186.e1.

33. Rastogi A, Puli S, El-Serag HB, et al. Incidence of esophageal adenocarcinoma in patients with Barrett's esophagus and high-grade dysplasia: a meta-analysis. Gastrointest Endosc 2008;67(3):394–8.

34. Titi M, Overhiser A, Ulusarac O, et al. Development of subsquamous high-grade dysplasia and adenocarcinoma after successful radiofrequency ablation of Barrett's esophagus. Gastroenterology 2012;143(3):564–6.e1.

35. Graham DY, Schwartz JT, Cain GD, et al. Prospective evaluation of biopsy number in the diagnosis of esophageal and gastric carcinoma. Gastroenterology 1982;82(2):228–31.

36. Network NCC. Esophageal and Esophagogastric Junction Cancers (Version 3.2015). Available at: http://www.nccn.org/professionals/physician_gls/pdf/esophageal.pdf. Accessed January 28, 2016.

37. Dunbar KB, Spechler SJ. The risk of lymph-node metastases in patients with high-grade dysplasia or intramucosal carcinoma in Barrett's esophagus: a systematic review. Am J Gastroenterol 2012;107(6):850–62 [quiz: 863].

38. Manner H, May A, Pech O, et al. Early Barrett's carcinoma with "low-risk" submucosal invasion: long-term results of endoscopic resection with a curative intent. Am J Gastroenterol 2008;103(10):2589–97.

39. Hur C, Miller M, Kong CY, et al. Trends in esophageal adenocarcinoma incidence and mortality. Cancer 2013;119(6):1149–58.

40. Larghi A, Lightdale CJ, Memeo L, et al. EUS followed by EMR for staging of high-grade dysplasia and early cancer in Barrett's esophagus. Gastrointest Endosc 2005;62(1):16–23.

41. Bruzzi JF, Munden RF, Truong MT, et al. PET/CT of esophageal cancer: its role in clinical management. Radiographics 2007;27(6):1635–52.

42. Puli SR, Reddy JB, Bechtold ML, et al. Staging accuracy of esophageal cancer by endoscopic ultrasound: a meta-analysis and systematic review. World J Gastroenterol 2008;14(10):1479–90.

43. Young PE, Gentry AB, Acosta RD, et al. Endoscopic ultrasound does not accurately stage early adenocarcinoma or high-grade dysplasia of the esophagus. Clin Gastroenterol Hepatol 2010;8(12):1037–41.
44. Pech O, May A, Manner H, et al. Long-term efficacy and safety of endoscopic resection for patients with mucosal adenocarcinoma of the esophagus. Gastroenterology 2014;146(3):652–60.e1.
45. Rubenstein JH, Shaheen NJ. Epidemiology, diagnosis, and management of esophageal adenocarcinoma. Gastroenterology 2015;149(2):302–17.e1.
46. Tsujii Y, Nishida T, Nishiyama O, et al. Clinical outcomes of endoscopic submucosal dissection for superficial esophageal neoplasms: a multicenter retrospective cohort study. Endoscopy 2015;47(9):775–83.
47. Shaheen NJ, Sharma P, Overholt BF, et al. Radiofrequency ablation in Barrett's esophagus with dysplasia. N Engl J Med 2009;360(22):2277–88.
48. Pasricha S, Bulsiewicz WJ, Hathorn KE, et al. Durability and predictors of successful radiofrequency ablation for Barrett's esophagus. Clin Gastroenterol Hepatol 2014;12(11):1840–7.e1.
49. Pech O, Bollschweiler E, Manner H, et al. Comparison between endoscopic and surgical resection of mucosal esophageal adenocarcinoma in Barrett's esophagus at two high-volume centers. Ann Surg 2011;254(1):67–72.
50. Napier KJ, Scheerer M, Misra S. Esophageal cancer: a review of epidemiology, pathogenesis, staging workup and treatment modalities. World J Gastrointest Oncol 2014;6(5):112–20.
51. Ardalan B, Spector SA, Livingstone AS, et al. Neoadjuvant, surgery and adjuvant chemotherapy without radiation for esophageal cancer. Jpn J Clin Oncol 2007; 37(8):590–6.
52. Oppedijk V, van der Gaast A, van Lanschot JJ, et al. Patterns of recurrence after surgery alone versus preoperative chemoradiotherapy and surgery in the CROSS trials. J Clin Oncol 2014;32(5):385–91.
53. Stahl M, Stuschke M, Lehmann N, et al. Chemoradiation with and without surgery in patients with locally advanced squamous cell carcinoma of the esophagus. J Clin Oncol 2005;23(10):2310–7.
54. Seiwert TY, Salama JK, Vokes EE. The concurrent chemoradiation paradigm–general principles. Nat Clin Pract Oncol 2007;4(2):86–100.
55. Cunningham D, Starling N, Rao S, et al. Capecitabine and oxaliplatin for advanced esophagogastric cancer. N Engl J Med 2008;358(1):36–46.
56. Chau I, Norman AR, Cunningham D, et al. Multivariate prognostic factor analysis in locally advanced and metastatic esophago-gastric cancer–pooled analysis from three multicenter, randomized, controlled trials using individual patient data. J Clin Oncol 2004;22(12):2395–403.
57. Knyrim K, Wagner HJ, Bethge N, et al. A controlled trial of an expansile metal stent for palliation of esophageal obstruction due to inoperable cancer. N Engl J Med 1993;329(18):1302–7.
58. Vennalaganti PR, Naag Kanakadandi V, Gross SA, et al. Inter-observer agreement among pathologists using wide-area transepithelial sampling with computer-assisted analysis in patients with Barrett's esophagus. Am J Gastroenterol 2015;110(9):1257–60.
59. Johanson JF, Frakes J, Eisen D, et al. Computer-assisted analysis of abrasive transepithelial brush biopsies increases the effectiveness of esophageal screening: a multicenter prospective clinical trial by the EndoCDx Collaborative Group. Dig Dis Sci 2011;56(3):767–72.

60. Sharma P, Bergman JJ, Goda K, et al. Development and validation of a classification system to identify high-grade dysplasia and esophageal adenocarcinoma in Barrett's esophagus using narrow band imaging. Gastroenterology 2016; 150(3):591–8.
61. Muto M, Minashi K, Yano T, et al. Early detection of superficial squamous cell carcinoma in the head and neck region and esophagus by narrow band imaging: a multicenter randomized controlled trial. J Clin Oncol 2010;28(9):1566–72.
62. Wang KK, Carr-Locke DL, Singh SK, et al. Use of probe-based confocal laser endomicroscopy (pCLE) in gastrointestinal applications. A consensus report based on clinical evidence. United European Gastroenterol J 2015;3(3):230–54.
63. Wolfsen HC, Sharma P, Wallace MB, et al. Safety and feasibility of volumetric laser endomicroscopy in patients with Barrett's esophagus (with videos). Gastrointest Endosc 2015;82(4):631–40.

# Current Perspectives on Gastric Cancer

 CrossMark

Juan M. Marqués-Lespier, MD[a], María González-Pons, PhD[b],
Marcia Cruz-Correa, MD, PhD[c],*

## KEYWORDS

- Gastric cancer • *Helicobacter pylori* • Atrophic gastritis • Intestinal metaplasia
- Dysplasia

## KEY POINTS

- Although gastric cancer (GC) incidence has declined in the United States during the last decade, an increase in the incidence of GC has been estimated for 2016.
- GC prognosis is very poor. Only 28.3% of newly discovered GCs are expected to survive longer than 5 years after diagnosis.
- Prognosis of GC is largely depends on the tumor stage at diagnosis and classification as intestinal or diffuse.
- Although nonsteroidal anti-inflammatory drugs, aspirins, and statins are reported to decrease GC risk, these have not been implemented for GC chemoprevention in clinical practice.
- Risk assessment and surveillance guidelines have been implemented in Asian countries with high incidence of GC. In the United States, only the American Society for Gastrointestinal Endoscopy has recently published guidelines for the screening and management gastric lesion.

## GLOBAL IMPACT OF GASTRIC CANCER

Despite the overall decrease in the incidence of gastric cancer (GC) since the 1930s, it is still a major cause of morbidity and mortality worldwide.[1] As many as 952,000 new GC cases were estimated in 2012 alone; making it the fifth most common incident cancer in the world and the third leading cause of cancer death in both sexes worldwide.[2] Among patients diagnosed with GC, close to 75% die from this disease.[3] GC also is responsible for 1 of the highest cancer burdens as determined by disability-adjusted life years lost.[4]

---

The authors have no conflicts of interest to disclose.
[a] Division of Gastroenterology, Department of Medicine, University of Puerto Rico School of Medicine, San Juan, PR 00935, USA; [b] University of Puerto Rico Comprehensive Cancer Center, San Juan, PR 00935, USA; [c] Departments of Medicine, Surgery, and Biochemistry, University of Puerto Rico, Medical Sciences Campus, San Juan, PR 00935, USA
* Corresponding author.
*E-mail address:* marcia.cruz1@upr.edu

Gastroenterol Clin N Am 45 (2016) 413–428
http://dx.doi.org/10.1016/j.gtc.2016.04.002
0889-8553/16/$ – see front matter © 2016 Elsevier Inc. All rights reserved.

**gastro.theclinics.com**

Globally, GC incidence has been shown to be more common in men and to increase with age, with most cases occurring after the age of 60 years.[2] However, GC incidence rates vary dramatically across countries. The geographic distribution of GC has been mainly attributed to differences in dietary patterns, socioeconomic status, and the prevalence of *Helicobacter pylori* infections.[5] The highest GC incidence and mortality rates occur in Eastern Asia, Central and Eastern Europe, and South America.[6] Mortality rates associated with GC, even in developed countries, are still very high; only 28.3% of newly diagnosed cases are expected to survive 5 years or longer after diagnosis.

According to the Surveillance, Epidemiology, and End Results Program, approximately 22,220 new GC cases were diagnosed in the United States (US) in 2014. An increase in the incidence of GC in the US has been estimated for 2016;[7] according to the American Cancer Society, approximately 26,370 individuals will be diagnosed with GC and 10,730 are expected to die due to this disease. Within the US, Hispanics, African Americans, and Native Americans are more frequently diagnosed with GC than non-Hispanic whites (**Fig. 1**).[3,8]

## GASTRIC CANCER CAUSES AND RISK FACTORS
### Infectious Agents Associated with Gastric Cancer

#### Helicobacter pylori

In 1994, the International Agency for Research on Cancer classified *H pylori*, the first formally recognized bacterial carcinogen, as a class I human carcinogen for GC. *H pylori* are involved in 90% of all gastric malignancies.[9] *H pylori* incidence varies according to age, ethnicity, and geographic location. In locations such as Mexico, Argentina, and Asian countries the prevalence of *H pylori* ranges from 30% to 70% by the age of 20 years and 70% to 90% by the age of 60 years. In the US and France, the prevalence is approximately 20% and 40% for younger and older ages, respectively.[10]

H pylori contributes to the development of gastric neoplasia by promoting inflammation in the gastric mucosa (gastritis), which leads to sequential histopathologic changes that may result in the development of GC (**Fig. 2**).[9,11] However, not every individual infected with *H pylori* will develop GC. The exact pathophysiological mechanisms, as well as the contribution of environmental risk factors and host genetic susceptibility in the progression of gastric carcinogenesis, have yet to be fully

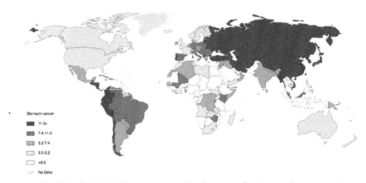

**Fig. 1.** Age-standardized GC incidence rates, both sexes for 2012. (*From* Ferlay J, Ervik M, Dikshit R, et al. GLOBOCAN 2012 v1.0, Cancer Incidence and Mortality Worldwide: IARC CancerBase No. 11. [Internet]. Lyon (France): International Agency for Research on Cancer; 2013. Available at: http://globocan.iarc.fr. Accessed October 11, 2014; with permission.)

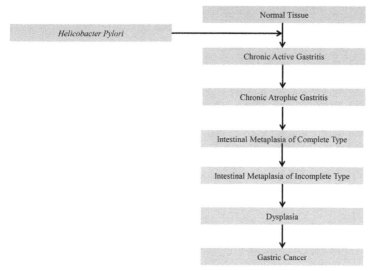

**Fig. 2.** The precancerous cascade. Prolonged gastric inflammation resulting from chronic *H pylori* infection causes epithelial damage that leads to gastric atrophy, characterized by loss of parietal cells and chief cells and glandular atrophy. The gastric epithelium is then replaced by intestinal metaplasia, followed by foci of low-grade dysplasia, which can later develop to high-grade dysplasia that can later become adenocarcinomas.

elucidated. *H pylori* virulence factors have been associated with a higher risk of GC. Infection with *H pylori* strains with *vacAs1-*, *vacAm1-*, and *cagA*-positive genotypes are associated with an approximate 6-fold increase in GC risk.[12] Increasing evidence supports that the extent of the inflammatory response to *H pylori* is in large part determined by polymorphisms in host genes encoding cytokines and cytokine receptors. Individuals with proinflammatory interleukin (IL)-1 genotypes infected with *H pylori* strains with *vacAs1-*, *vacAm1-*, and *cagA*-positive genotypes were reported to have up to an 87-fold higher risk of GC compared with *H pylori*-infected individuals without proinflammatory IL-1 polymorphisms.[13] Recently, GC stem cells were also proposed as a gastric carcinogenesis mechanism. Chronic infection with *H pylori* induces recruitment of bone marrow-derived cells that, once recruited, differentiate with local gastric epithelial cells, ultimately inducing stem cell properties and leading to cell metaplasia, dysplasia, and adenocarcinoma.[14] Unfortunately, there are currently no robust biomarkers clinically available to reliably predict who will develop GC cancer after *H pylori* infection.

### Epstein-Barr virus
Multiple studies in different parts of the world have found the prevalence of Epstein-Barr virus (EBV) in 5% to 16% of gastric carcinomas, which supports its possible role as an etiologic agent of GC.[15] In Asia, Europe, and the Americas, prevalence of EBV is close to 9% of all GC cases reported.[16] Male patients have been found to be twice as likely to have EBV-positive tumors compared with females. Tumors in the gastric cardia or corpus were found to be twice as likely to be EBV-positive compared with those in the antrum.[16] Although the role of EBV in gastric carcinogenesis is not yet clearly defined, EBV-positivity has been reported to be associated with favorable prognosis.[17]

### Genetic Predisposition: Familial Gastric Cancer

An estimated 20% of GC patients have a family history of GC.[18] According to the racial or ethnic group, family history was shown to confer 2-fold to 10-fold increased risk of GC.[19] Although most GCs are sporadic, 10% of the cases have familial clustering and 1% to 3% are hereditary.[20] Hereditary GC includes syndromes such as hereditary diffuse GC (HDGC), gastric adenocarcinoma and proximal polyposis of the stomach, and familial intestinal GC. HDGC is a rare, autosomal dominant disorder that is responsible for 1% to 3% of all familial GC cases.[21] About 40% of individuals with HDGC have germline mutations in the *CDH1* gene, which encodes E-cadherin.[22] In the presence of *CDH1* mutations, the lifetime risk of developing GC is 70% to 80%.[21] GC can also develop as part of familial cancer syndromes, including Lynch syndrome, familial adenomatous polyposis, Peutz-Jeghers syndrome, and Li-Fraumeni syndrome.[23] GC is part of the Lynch syndrome tumor spectrum; GC risk is 2.9 times higher for subjects with germline *MLH1* mutations.[24]

### Demographic, Environmental, and Lifestyle Risk Factors

In addition to infectious agents and family history, additional GC risk factors include age, gender, certain occupations, tobacco use, diet, and being overweight, among others. The risk of developing GC is twice as high in men as in women and it is usually diagnosed between the ages of 60 to 80 years. Individuals with certain occupations, such as those who work in the coal, metal, and rubber industries, have been reported to have an increased risk of GC.[25] Tobacco smoking has been reported to cause a 60% and 20% increase in GC risk in men and women, respectively.[26] It is estimated that 18% of GC cases are attributable to tobacco smoking.[27] No association has been found between smokeless tobacco and GC.[28] In contrast, alcohol consumption has not been consistently shown to be associated with GC; however, it has been identified as a risk factor for disease progression.[29] A 5-fold increased risk of GC has been observed as a result of the combined effect of alcohol and smoking.[30] A high intake of salted, pickled or smoked foods, and preserved foods rich in salt and nitrites have been reported to be associated with an increased risk of GC, whereas foods rich in fiber, vegetables, and fruit were found to be protective.[31] Individuals with moderate and high salt intake had a 1.41 and 1.68 relative risk (RR) for GC, respectively, compared with those who consumed low levels of salt.[32,33] Additionally, in the presence of *H pylori* infection, high salt intake further increases the risk of GC.[34,35] Significant associations were found between the consumption of processed meat (RR 1.45 95%, CI 1.26–1.65) and GC risk.[36] This association between processed meats and GC been described to be stronger in subjects infected with *H pylori*.[37] Although obesity has not been found to be associated to all GCs, several meta-analyses have reported a positive association between increased body mass index (BMI) and risk of GC in the cardia.[38]

## GASTRIC CANCER CLASSIFICATION

GC is classified into 2 main groups: early and advanced stages. Prognosis is largely depends on the tumor stage. The 5-year survival rate in patients with early GC (EGC) is between 85% and 100%, whereas it is only 5% to 20% for advanced GC.[39] The degree of invasion defines GC as early or advanced.[40] Early gastric carcinoma is defined as malignancies limited to the mucosa or submucosa, regardless of lymph node invasion. Advanced GC is classified according to the extent of invasion and endoscopic appearance (polypoid lesions, ulcerated with well-defined border, ulcerated with ill-defined borders, or infiltrating diffuse without evidence of mass or ulcers).

Tumor location dictates the anatomic classification as cardia or noncardia (distal from the cardia) (**Fig. 3**). Cardia and noncardia adenocarcinomas present with different clinical and epidemiologic characteristics.[21] In contrast to cardia tumors, noncardia tumors have decreased in the last decades. Cardia GC affects predominantly white populations and is more often associated with gastroesophageal reflux disease.[21] Cardia adenocarcinomas are aggressive and have a poor prognosis. Cardia tumors invade the gastric and esophageal walls and metastasize to local lymph nodes (**Table 1**). Due their aggressiveness, the American Joint Classification of Cancer decided to use the esophageal cancer staging system for all GC arising in the esophagogastric junction and any cancer arising in the proximal 5 cm of the stomach with involvement of the esophagogastric junction.[44] Noncardia GC is more likely associated with *H pylori* and comprises more than 60% all GC cases worldwide.[45]

### Histologic Classification

The Lauren classification system,[46] which classifies GC as intestinal (with intercellular junctions) and diffuse (without intercellular junctions), is the most frequently used system to classify GC (see **Table 1**). Intestinal-type adenocarcinomas form glands or tubules lined by epithelium, resembling the intestinal mucosa. Although the incidence of intestinal-type GC has decreased recently, it is still the most frequent type of GC found in high incidence populations.[21] This type of GC usually occurs in a 2:1 male-to-female ratio and in individuals between 55 and 80 years of age.[42] The development of intestinal-type GC is preceded by a sequence of histologic lesions that my take years to develop (see **Fig. 2**).[47]

Diffuse-type gastric adenocarcinomas are more aggressive and have a worse prognosis than intestinal-type. They do not have a gender bias and are generally diagnosed

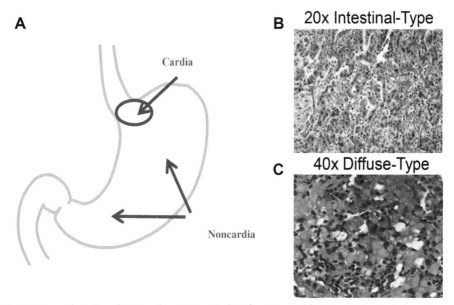

**Fig. 3.** Tumor location dictates the anatomic classification and histopathological characteristics. (*A*) GC classification according to anatomic locations. (*B*) Hematoxylin-eosin, original magnification ×20, intestinal-type noncardia GC. (*C*) Hematoxylin-eosin, original magnification ×40, diffuse-type noncardia GC. (*Courtesy of* Dr Carmen Gonzalez Keelan, San Juan, Puerto Rico.)

Table 1
Gastric cancer characteristics according to location and classification

| Cardia Gastric Cancer | Noncardia Gastric Cancer | |
| --- | --- | --- |
| | Intestinal-Type | Diffuse-Type |
| • Incidence is increasing[41]<br>• Associated with gastro-esophageal reflux<br>• Resembles esophageal adenocarcinoma[41]<br>• More aggressive and worse prognosis than noncardia[41]<br>• Associated with white population and strong male predominance (6:1)[41] | • Incidence is decreasing[21,42]<br>• Associated with H pylori[21]<br>• Presents with precancerous lesions[43]<br>• Histologic characteristics: malignant epithelial cells and hyperchromatic irregular and angulated glands that show cohesiveness and glandular differentiation infiltrating the stroma<br>• May present in 3 scenarios: polypoid lesion attached on a wide base, an ulcerated carcinoma with sharp and raised margins, and an ulcerated carcinoma without definite limits[21]<br>• Diagnosed in individuals ages 55–80 y[42]<br>• Male to female ratio 2:1[42] | • Incidence is increasing[8]<br>• Can be associated with H pylori, strongly associated with loss of expression of E-cadherin[43]<br>• No precancerous lesions[43]<br>• Histologic characteristics: cells lacking cohesion invading tissues independently or in small clusters<br>• Lesions are nonulcerated, diffusely infiltrating carcinomas<br>• Signet ring adenocarcinoma: variant of the diffuse histologic type with abundant cytoplasmic mucin that displaces the nucleus to the periphery[8,21]<br>• Diagnosed in younger patients ages 40–60 y[8,21]<br>• Male to female ratio 1:1[42]<br>• Worst prognosis than intestinal-type GC[8]<br>• HDGC autosomal dominant pattern of inheritance[43] |

in younger patients (40–60 years of age). Diffuse GC cells lack cohesion, and invade tissues independently or in small clusters.[8] A variant of the diffuse histologic type is the signet ring cell gastric adenocarcinoma. Signet tumor cells contain abundant cytoplasmic mucin that displaces the nucleus toward the periphery.[8,21] Although diffuse-type GC can be associated with H pylori infections, it is more frequently associated with loss of expression of E-cadherin (HDGC); no precancerous lesions have been defined to date.[43]

## GASTRIC CANCER PREVENTION
### Lifestyle Modification

Primary prevention aims to prevent the disease before it ever occurs by preventing exposures to hazards, changing unhealthy or unsafe behaviors, and increasing resistance to the disease. Recommended lifestyle changes to prevent GC include limiting exposure to tobacco and maintaining a healthy BMI. In terms of diet, consumption of fresh fruit and vegetables 1 or more days per week significantly reduces GC risk, as demonstrated in numerous prospective studies.[48] Consumption of antioxidants has also been recommended for the prevention of GC; however, some clinical trials have conflicting results.[39,49]

## Chemoprevention

Cyclooxygenase (COX)-2 overexpression is characteristic of noncardia stomach cancers and in well-differentiated stomach cancers,[50] suggesting that suppression of COX-2 could be used as a chemopreventive strategy to prevent GC. Several cohort and observational studies have suggested that systematic use of nonaspirin nonsteroidal anti-inflammatory drugs (NSAIDs) and aspirin are protective factors, especially for noncardia GC with *H pylori* infection.[51,52] However, randomized controlled trials evaluating the role of nonaspirin NSAIDs for regression of intestinal metaplasia (IM) after eradication of *H pylori* failed to demonstrate a benefit compared with individuals without nonaspirin NSAID use.[53,54] The use of celecoxib, a nonaspirin NSAID, has been shown to regress precancerous stomach mucosal conditions and/or lesions after *H pylori* eradication.[55] Statins are associated with a significant decrease in GC risk and have also been studied as potential GC chemopreventive agents.[56]

## Helicobacter pylori Eradication

Because only a very small proportion of *H pylori*-infected subjects develop GC, the benefit of mass *H pylori* eradication campaigns to prevent GC remains unsubstantiated.[57] However, treatment and eradication of *H pylori* infection is recommended in patients with gastritis. *H pylori* eradication has been reported to restore gastric histology to normal in individuals with chronic gastritis and atrophic gastritis without IM.[58] Atrophic gastritis has been reported to undergo regression within 1 or 2 years after successful eradication of *H pylori*.[59] The presence of IM in *H pylori*-associated chronic gastritis suggests a less reversible stage compared with atrophic gastritis alone. Evidence suggests that eradication at the IM stage is less effective and that lesions are more likely to progress.[60] In a randomized 6-year follow-up clinical trial examining the role of anti-*H pylori* treatment and dietary antioxidant micronutrient supplementation in reducing the progression of precancerous lesions, use of anti-*H pylori* treatment or antioxidants was associated with significant inhibition of precancerous lesions including IM.[39] This reversion of gastric atrophy and IM was confirmed after 12 years.[61] The eradication of *H pylori* in GC patients with prior endoscopic resection reduces the incidence of new tumors and the extent of IM.[62] There are controversial data regarding the effect of *H pylori* eradication on the development of gastric epithelial dysplasia.[63] At present, prophylactic *H pylori* eradication is strongly recommended after endoscopic tumor resection in EGC to prevent recurrence of malignancy.[64]

## SCREENING AND SURVEILLANCE

Because GC can take decades to develop, the identification of precancerous lesions and endoscopic surveillance of patients at high risk may help to detect early-stage malignancies when they are still operable and have better prognosis. In a large-scale 10-year follow-up study, progression rates to GC for subjects with atrophic gastritis, IM, low-grade dysplasia, or high-grade dysplasia were estimated 0.8%, 1.8%, 4.0% and 33.0%, respectively.[65] Therefore, there is insufficient evidence to conclude that it would be beneficial and cost-effective to implement population GC screening in regions not at high risk of GC. It has been suggested that the GC screening strategy should be based on GC incidence in the population and on the individual's risk.

Asian countries (Japan, South Korea, Singapore, and Taiwan), which have a high incidence of GC, have started national screening programs. The Korean National Cancer Screening Program (NCSP) provides regular 2-year interval GC screening by upper gastrointestinal radiograph or upper endoscopy for citizens aged 40 years or older.[66]

The current trend in GC mortality reduction, despite the stable age-standardized GC incidence during last decade, supports that the current screening program has a mortality-reducing effect in Korea.[67] However, the current Korean NCSP does not recommend different screening intervals depending on pre-existing gastric lesions for risk stratification. In Japan, guidelines for GC screening recommend photofluorography (indirect radiograph using small films) for population-based and opportunistic screening.[68] They do not recommend endoscopy as a screening tool in the general population due to the lack of sufficient evidence supporting a reduction of GC as a result of population endoscopy screening.

The European Society of Gastrointestinal Endoscopy, a group of European gastrological societies, recently published management of precancerous conditions and lesions in the stomach (MAPS) guidelines for high-risk groups (**Table 2**).[69] These guidelines emphasize the importance of GC risk stratification. The application of the operative link on gastritis assessment (OLGA) and operative link for gastric IM (OLGIM) to address the grade and extension of atrophy may be useful for identifying subgroups of patients with risk of progression to GC.[71,72] Both OLGA and OLGIM have been validated in prospective studies.[73,74] In the US, only the American Society for Gastrointestinal Endoscopy (ASGE) has recently published guidelines for the screening and management gastric lesions based on MAPS (see **Table 2**).[70]

**Table 2**
**Surveillance guidelines for precancerous conditions and lesions in the stomach**

| Premalignant Lesion | European Society of Gastrointestinal Endoscopy (MAPS) Guidelines[69] | American Society for Gastrointestinal Endoscopy Guidelines[70] |
|---|---|---|
| Atrophic Gastritis or IM | • At least 4 nontarget biopsies from 2 topographic sites should be taken for adequate staging and grading of the premalignant condition<br>• Patients with extensive atrophy and/or IM should be offered endoscopic surveillance<br>• A 3-y follow-up after diagnosis is recommended for patients with extensive atrophy and/or IM<br>• Surveillance endoscopy is not recommended for patients with mild to moderate atrophy and/or IM restricted to stomach antrum | • A surveillance endoscopy for patients with GIM who are at increased risk of GC (Asian ethnicity or family history of GC)<br>• Surveillance intervals should be individualized |
| Low-Grade Dysplasia | • In the absence of an endoscopically defined lesion, follow-up within 1 y<br>• In the presence of endoscopically defined lesion, consider endoscopic resection obtain a more accurate histologic diagnosis | • A follow-up EGD within 1 y with a topographic mapping biopsy strategy is indicated |
| High-Grade Dysplasia | • In the absence of endoscopically defined lesions, immediate endoscopic reassessment with extensive biopsy sampling and surveillance at 6-mo to 1-y intervals is indicated | • Endoscopic resection and surveillance endoscopy is recommended |

Studies suggest that individuals with GC family history do not necessarily need more frequent GC screening than the generally recommended 2-year interval in Korea.[18] Recommendations for management and surveillance of familial GC have only been made for individuals with HDGC.[75] A prophylactic gastrectomy is recommended to those having a *CDH1* mutation at about 20 years of age; however, annual endoscopic surveillance using a high-definition endoscope should be offered for those who do not have a gastrectomy.[76] *H pylori* treatment is recommended by European and Chinese guidelines for the first-degree family members of GC patients[77]; however, the 2008 version of the Japanese guidelines did not recommend treatment due to lack of direct evidence of GC prevention in family members.[78]

## DIAGNOSTIC EVALUATION

Endoscopic diagnosis of GC may be difficult because EGC often only shows only minimal, subtle changes in the gastric mucosa. The first step in diagnosing GC endoscopically is to detect any suspicious lesions and to characterize them. Good reporting based on the Paris classification as the current standard is imperative.[79] The European Society of Gastrointestinal Endoscopy recommends that, for quality control, 8 images should be taken to illustrate the examination of the stomach in its totality (complementary images should be taken in the case of a specific lesion).[80] Detection of subtle gastric mucosal changes during examination requires the use advanced endoscopic techniques, such as narrow-band imaging (NBI) or magnifying endoscopy with NBI (NBI-ME), which has high sensitivity and specificity.[80,81] NBI endoscopy may also help in assessing the extent of the lesions, and in improving safety margins and cure rates during endoscopic resection of EGC. Other techniques, including chromoendoscopy, flexible spectral imaging color enhancement endoscopy with or without magnification, and confocal laser endomicroscopy, have shown promising results.[82–84] At present, NBI-ME is probably the most frequently used endoscopic technique and has the largest amount of technical data available.

Endoscopic training and experience is essential, as well as good preparation for the endoscopic examination, for the diagnosis of GC. The most important process in the endoscopic diagnosis of GC is the scrutiny all gastric areas with targeted biopsies because histopathological examination remains the gold standard for the final diagnosis.[85] Generally, the mass or abnormal mucosa is targeted for biopsy. In the case of a malignant gastric ulcer, at least 7 biopsies of the heaped up edges of the ulcer and base should be performed.[86] Diagnosis of linitis plastica can be more difficult due to reduction in the yield of mucosal biopsies. Large mucosal and submucosal biopsy samples may be taken with snare resection. Endoscopic ultrasound with fine-needle aspiration or core sampling may be necessary but histopathology is still generally preferable to cytology for diagnosis.[70]

## CLINICAL MANAGEMENT

Guidelines in Europe[87] and the US[88] have been proposed for management of GC depending on location, stage, and surgical candidacy. GC screening in countries with high-risk populations is effective in identifying EGC, which can be treated endoscopically. Accurate pretreatment staging is critical in identifying EGC patients with disease that is limited to the mucosa and submucosa (stage T1) and who are candidates for endoscopic mucosal resection (EMR) or endoscopic submucosal dissection (ESD).[89] ESD permits en bloc resection of most lesions and is the preferred technique for resecting EGC in Asia,[90] with a complete en bloc resection rate of 87.7% and low complication rates.[91] ESD has been reported to outperform EMR for en bloc, complete, and curative resection with lower recurrence rate.[92] In the US, ESD is rarely performed outside referral centers with expertise in this technique.[70] Depending on the size and location of the primary tumor, the preferred means of therapy is surgical resection with total or subtotal gastrectomy.[93]

Although several targeted therapies have been studied, only 2 targeted GC treatments have been approved for use in the US. Inhibition of human growth factor receptor 2 (HER2) has been tested as a targeted therapy for several cancers, including GC. Trastuzumab is a monoclonal antibody that targets HER2 that inhibits HER2-mediated signaling, and thereby prevents the proliferation of HER2-dependent tumors.[94] The trastuzumab for gastric cancer (ToGA) trial, a phase III international study evaluating the efficacy of trastuzumab in combination with conventional therapy (cisplatin plus 5-fluorouracil or capecitabine), showed improvement in the overall survival compared with chemotherapy alone.[95] Ramucirumab, a human monoclonal antibody against the vascular endothelial growth factor receptor 2 (an important signaling pathway in GC and gastroesophageal cancer), is the first biologic therapy approved by the US Food and Drug Administration used as a single agent that demonstrates survival benefit in patients with advanced GC or gastroesophageal cancer who have progressed after first-line treatment.[96]

## PROGNOSIS AND SURVIVORSHIP

In the US, relative 5-year survival rates for GC increased from 15% to 29% from 1975 to 2009.[97] However, GC survival remains poor. Cardia GC and diffuse-type noncardia GC present with the worst prognosis.[8,41] Compared with tumors in the pyloric antrum, cardia GC have lower 5-year survival and higher operative mortality.[98] Overall, EGC can be associated with 5-year survival rates that approximate 90%. However, in both the US and Europe, few cancers are detected at early stages, resulting in the low 5-year relative survival rates.[99,100] This emphasizes the importance of implementing public health measures that help identify individuals at high risk to increase early diagnosis and decrease GC mortality.

## ACKNOWLEDGMENTS

We would like to thank Dr. Carmen Gonzalez-Keelan, Professor at the Department of Pathology at the University of Puerto Rico, for providing the histology images. This project was supported by the Puerto Rico Clinical and Translational Research Consortium (award number U54MD007587) from the National Institute on Minority Health and Health Disparities and by the UPR/MDACC Partnership for Excellence in Cancer Research Program (award number U54 CA096297) from the National Cancer Institute. The content is solely the responsibility of the authors and does not necessarily represent the official views of the National Institutes of Health.

## REFERENCES

1. Kelley JR, Duggan JM. Gastric cancer epidemiology and risk factors. J Clin Epidemiol 2003;56(1):1–9.
2. Ferlay J, Soerjomataram I, Dikshit R, et al. Cancer incidence and mortality worldwide: sources, methods and major patterns in GLOBOCAN 2012. Int J Cancer 2015;136(5):E359–86.
3. Ferlay J, Shin HR, Bray F, et al. Estimates of worldwide burden of cancer in 2008: GLOBOCAN 2008. Int J Cancer 2010;127(12):2893–917.

4. Soerjomataram I, Lortet-Tieulent J, Parkin DM, et al. Global burden of cancer in 2008: a systematic analysis of disability-adjusted life-years in 12 world regions. Lancet 2012;380(9856):1840–50.
5. Jemal A, Bray F, Center MM, et al. Global cancer statistics. CA Cancer J Clin 2011;61(2):69–90.
6. Ferlay J, Soerjomataram I, Ervik M, et al. GLOBOCAN 2012 v1.0, Cancer incidence and mortality Worldwide: IARC CancerBase No. 11 [Internet]. Lyon (France): International Agency for Research on Cancer; 2013. Available at: http://globocan.iarc.fr. Accessed October 11, 2014.
7. American Cancer Society. Cancer Facts & Figures 2016. Atlanta (GA): American Cancer Society; 2016.
8. Correa P. Gastric cancer: overview. Gastroenterol Clin North Am 2013;42(2): 211–7.
9. Noto JM, Peek RM Jr. *Helicobacter pylori*: an overview. Methods Mol Biol 2012; 921:7–10.
10. Pounder RE, Ng D. The prevalence of *Helicobacter pylori* infection in different countries. Aliment Pharmacol Ther 1995;9(Suppl 2):33–9.
11. Correa P, Cuello C, Duque E. Carcinoma and intestinal metaplasia of the stomach in Colombian migrants. J Natl Cancer Inst 1970;44(2):297–306.
12. An international association between *Helicobacter pylori* infection and gastric cancer. The EUROGAST Study Group. Lancet 1993;341(8857):1359–62.
13. Figueiredo C, Machado JC, Pharoah P, et al. *Helicobacter pylori* and interleukin 1 genotyping: an opportunity to identify high-risk individuals for gastric carcinoma. J Natl Cancer Inst 2002;94(22):1680–7.
14. Bessede E, Dubus P, Megraud F, et al. *Helicobacter pylori* infection and stem cells at the origin of gastric cancer. Oncogene 2015;34(20):2547–55.
15. Chen XZ, Chen H, Castro FA, et al. Epstein-Barr virus infection and gastric cancer: a systematic review. Medicine (Baltimore) 2015;94(20):e792.
16. Murphy G, Pfeiffer R, Camargo MC, et al. Meta-analysis shows that prevalence of Epstein-Barr virus-positive gastric cancer differs based on sex and anatomic location. Gastroenterology 2009;137(3):824–33.
17. Camargo MC, Kim WH, Chiaravalli AM, et al. Improved survival of gastric cancer with tumour Epstein-Barr virus positivity: an international pooled analysis. Gut 2014;63(2):236–43.
18. Han MA, Oh MG, Choi IJ, et al. Association of family history with cancer recurrence and survival in patients with gastric cancer. J Clin Oncol 2012;30(7): 701–8.
19. Yaghoobi M, Bijarchi R, Narod SA. Family history and the risk of gastric cancer. Br J Cancer 2010;102(2):237–42.
20. Figueiredo C, Costa S, Karameris A, et al. Pathogenesis of gastric cancer. Helicobacter 2015;20(Suppl 1):30–5.
21. Piazuelo MB, Correa P. Gastric cancer: overview. Colomb Med (Cali) 2013; 44(3):192–201.
22. Oliveira C, Pinheiro H, Figueiredo J, et al. Familial gastric cancer: genetic susceptibility, pathology, and implications for management. Lancet Oncol 2015; 16(2):e60–70.
23. Oliveira C, Seruca R, Carneiro F. Genetics, pathology, and clinics of familial gastric cancer. Int J Surg Pathol 2006;14(1):21–33.
24. Capelle LG, Van Grieken NC, Lingsma HF, et al. Risk and epidemiological time trends of gastric cancer in Lynch syndrome carriers in the Netherlands. Gastroenterology 2010;138(2):487–92.

25. Raj A, Mayberry JF, Podas T. Occupation and gastric cancer. Postgrad Med J 2003;79(931):252–8.
26. Ladeiras-Lopes R, Pereira AK, Nogueira A, et al. Smoking and gastric cancer: systematic review and meta-analysis of cohort studies. Cancer Causes Control 2008;19(7):689–701.
27. Gonzalez CA, Pera G, Agudo A, et al. Smoking and the risk of gastric cancer in the European Prospective Investigation Into Cancer and Nutrition (EPIC). Int J Cancer 2003;107(4):629–34.
28. Sinha DN, Abdulkader RS, Gupta PC. Smokeless tobacco-associated cancers: a systematic review and meta-analysis of Indian studies. Int J Cancer 2016; 138(6):1368–79.
29. Leung WK, Lin SR, Ching JY, et al. Factors predicting progression of gastric intestinal metaplasia: results of a randomised trial on *Helicobacter pylori* eradication. Gut 2004;53(9):1244–9.
30. Sjodahl K, Lu Y, Nilsen TI, et al. Smoking and alcohol drinking in relation to risk of gastric cancer: a population-based, prospective cohort study. Int J Cancer 2007;120(1):128–32.
31. Abnet CC, Corley DA, Freedman ND, et al. Diet and upper gastrointestinal malignancies. Gastroenterology 2015;148(6):1234–43.e4.
32. D'Elia L, Rossi G, Ippolito R, et al. Habitual salt intake and risk of gastric cancer: a meta-analysis of prospective studies. Clin Nutr 2012;31(4):489–98.
33. Ge S, Feng X, Shen L, et al. Association between habitual dietary salt intake and risk of gastric cancer: a systematic review of observational studies. Gastroenterol Res Pract 2012;2012:808120.
34. de Martel C, Forman D, Plummer M. Gastric cancer: epidemiology and risk factors. Gastroenterol Clin North Am 2013;42(2):219–40.
35. Peleteiro B, Lopes C, Figueiredo C, et al. Salt intake and gastric cancer risk according *to Helicobacter pylori* infection, smoking, tumour site and histological type. Br J Cancer 2011;104(1):198–207.
36. Zhu H, Yang X, Zhang C, et al. Red and processed meat intake is associated with higher gastric cancer risk: a meta-analysis of epidemiological observational studies. PLoS One 2013;8(8):e70955.
37. Gonzalez CA, Agudo A. Carcinogenesis, prevention and early detection of gastric cancer: where we are and where we should go. Int J Cancer 2012; 130(4):745–53.
38. Chen Y, Liu L, Wang X, et al. Body mass index and risk of gastric cancer: a meta-analysis of a population with more than ten million from 24 prospective studies. Cancer Epidemiol Biomarkers Prev 2013;22(8):1395–408.
39. Correa P, Fontham ET, Bravo JC, et al. Chemoprevention of gastric dysplasia: randomized trial of antioxidant supplements and anti-*Helicobacter pylori* therapy. J Natl Cancer Inst 2000;92(23):1881–8.
40. Japanese Gastric Cancer Association. Japanese classification of gastric carcinoma: 3rd English edition. Gastric Cancer 2011;14(2):101–12.
41. Botterweck AA, Schouten LJ, Volovics A, et al. Trends in incidence of adenocarcinoma of the oesophagus and gastric cardia in ten European countries. Int J Epidemiol 2000;29(4):645–54.
42. Henson DE, Dittus C, Younes M, et al. Differential trends in the intestinal and diffuse types of gastric carcinoma in the United States, 1973-2000: increase in the signet ring cell type. Arch Pathol Lab Med 2004;128(7):765–70.
43. Barber M, Murrell A, Ito Y, et al. Mechanisms and sequelae of E-cadherin silencing in hereditary diffuse gastric cancer. J Pathol 2008;216(3):295–306.

44. Washington K. 7th edition of the AJCC cancer staging manual: stomach. Ann Surg Oncol 2010;17(12):3077–9.
45. Colquhoun A, Arnold M, Ferlay J, et al. Global patterns of cardia and non-cardia gastric cancer incidence in 2012. Gut 2015;64(12):1881–8.
46. Lauren P. The two histological main types of gastric carcinoma: diffuse and so-called intestinal-type carcinoma. An attempt at a histo-clinical classification. Acta Pathol Microbiol Scand 1965;64:31–49.
47. Correa P, Cuello C, Duque E, et al. Gastric cancer in Colombia. III. Natural history of precursor lesions. J Natl Cancer Inst 1976;57(5):1027–35.
48. Kobayashi M, Tsubono Y, Sasazuki S, et al. Vegetables, fruit and risk of gastric cancer in Japan: a 10-year follow-up of the JPHC Study Cohort I. Int J Cancer 2002;102(1):39–44.
49. Plummer M, Vivas J, Lopez G, et al. Chemoprevention of precancerous gastric lesions with antioxidant vitamin supplementation: a randomized trial in a high-risk population. J Natl Cancer Inst 2007;99(2):137–46.
50. Song J, Su H, Zhou YY, et al. Cyclooxygenase-2 expression is associated with poor overall survival of patients with gastric cancer: a meta-analysis. Dig Dis Sci 2014;59(2):436–45.
51. Wu CY, Wu MS, Kuo KN, et al. Effective reduction of gastric cancer risk with regular use of nonsteroidal anti-inflammatory drugs in *Helicobacter pylori*-infected patients. J Clin Oncol 2010;28(18):2952–7.
52. Tian W, Zhao Y, Liu S, et al. Meta-analysis on the relationship between nonsteroidal anti-inflammatory drug use and gastric cancer. Eur J Cancer Prev 2010; 19(4):288–98.
53. Leung WK, Ng EK, Chan FK, et al. Effects of long-term rofecoxib on gastric intestinal metaplasia: results of a randomized controlled trial. Clin Cancer Res 2006;12(15):4766–72.
54. Yanaoka K, Oka M, Yoshimura N, et al. Preventive effects of etodolac, a selective cyclooxygenase-2 inhibitor, on cancer development in extensive metaplastic gastritis, a *Helicobacter pylori*-negative precancerous lesion. Int J Cancer 2010;126(6):1467–73.
55. Hung KH, Yang HB, Cheng HC, et al. Short-term celecoxib to regress long-term persistent gastric intestinal metaplasia after *Helicobacter pylori* eradication. J Gastroenterol Hepatol 2010;25(1):48–53.
56. Singh PP, Singh S. Statins are associated with reduced risk of gastric cancer: a systematic review and meta-analysis. Ann Oncol 2013;24(7):1721–30.
57. Compare D, Rocco A, Nardone G. Screening for and surveillance of gastric cancer. World J Gastroenterol 2014;20(38):13681–91.
58. Rokkas T, Pistiolas D, Sechopoulos P, et al. The long-term impact of *Helicobacter pylori* eradication on gastric histology: a systematic review and meta-analysis. Helicobacter 2007;12(Suppl 2):32–8.
59. De Vries AC, Kuipers EJ. Review article: *Helicobacter pylori* eradication for the prevention of gastric cancer. Aliment Pharmacol Ther 2007;26(Suppl 2):25–35.
60. Wang J, Xu L, Shi R, et al. Gastric atrophy and intestinal metaplasia before and after *Helicobacter pylori* eradication: a meta-analysis. Digestion 2011;83(4): 253–60.
61. Mera R, Fontham ET, Bravo LE, et al. Long term follow up of patients treated for *Helicobacter pylori* infection. Gut 2005;54(11):1536–40.
62. Uemura N, Mukai T, Okamoto S, et al. Effect of *Helicobacter pylori* eradication on subsequent development of cancer after endoscopic resection of early gastric cancer. Cancer Epidemiol Biomarkers Prev 1997;6(8):639–42.

63. You WC, Brown LM, Zhang L, et al. Randomized double-blind factorial trial of three treatments to reduce the prevalence of precancerous gastric lesions. J Natl Cancer Inst 2006;98(14):974–83.

64. Fukase K, Kato M, Kikuchi S, et al. Effect of eradication of *Helicobacter pylori* on incidence of metachronous gastric carcinoma after endoscopic resection of early gastric cancer: an open-label, randomised controlled trial. Lancet 2008;372(9636):392–7.

65. de Vries AC, van Grieken NC, Looman CW, et al. Gastric cancer risk in patients with premalignant gastric lesions: a nationwide cohort study in the Netherlands. Gastroenterology 2008;134(4):945–52.

66. Lee KS, Oh DK, Han MA, et al. Gastric cancer screening in Korea: report on the national cancer screening program in 2008. Cancer Res Treat 2011;43(2):83–8.

67. Jung KW, Won YJ, Kong HJ, et al. Cancer statistics in Korea: incidence, mortality, survival, and prevalence in 2011. Cancer Res Treat 2014;46(2):109–23.

68. Hamashima C, Shibuya D, Yamazaki H, et al. The Japanese guidelines for gastric cancer screening. Jpn J Clin Oncol 2008;38(4):259–67.

69. Dinis-Ribeiro M, Areia M, de Vries AC, et al. Management of precancerous conditions and lesions in the stomach (MAPS): guideline from the European Society of Gastrointestinal Endoscopy (ESGE), European Helicobacter Study Group (EHSG), European Society of Pathology (ESP), and the Sociedade Portuguesa de Endoscopia Digestiva (SPED). Endoscopy 2012;44(1):74–94.

70. ASGE Standards of Practice Committee, Evans JA, Chandrasekhara V, et al. The role of endoscopy in the management of premalignant and malignant conditions of the stomach. Gastrointest Endosc 2015;82(1):1–8.

71. Rugge M, Genta RM. Staging gastritis: an international proposal. Gastroenterology 2005;129(5):1807–8.

72. Capelle LG, de Vries AC, Haringsma J, et al. The staging of gastritis with the OLGA system by using intestinal metaplasia as an accurate alternative for atrophic gastritis. Gastrointest Endosc 2010;71(7):1150–8.

73. Satoh K, Osawa H, Yoshizawa M, et al. Assessment of atrophic gastritis using the OLGA system. Helicobacter 2008;13(3):225–9.

74. Rugge M, de Boni M, Pennelli G, et al. Gastritis OLGA-staging and gastric cancer risk: a twelve-year clinico-pathological follow-up study. Aliment Pharmacol Ther 2010;31(10):1104–11.

75. Choi IJ. Endoscopic gastric cancer screening and surveillance in high-risk groups. Clin Endosc 2014;47(6):497–503.

76. Kluijt I, Sijmons RH, Hoogerbrugge N, et al. Familial gastric cancer: guidelines for diagnosis, treatment and periodic surveillance. Fam Cancer 2012;11(3): 363–9.

77. Liu WZ, Xie Y, Cheng H, et al. Fourth Chinese National Consensus Report on the management of *Helicobacter pylori* infection. J Dig Dis 2013;14(5):211–21.

78. Asaka M, Kato M, Takahashi S, et al. Guidelines for the management of *Helicobacter pylori* infection in Japan: 2009 revised edition. Helicobacter 2010;15(1): 1–20.

79. The Paris endoscopic classification of superficial neoplastic lesions: esophagus, stomach, and colon: November 30 to December 1, 2002. Gastrointest Endosc 2003;58(6 Suppl):S3–43.

80. Rey JF, Lambert R. ESGE recommendations for quality control in gastrointestinal endoscopy: guidelines for image documentation in upper and lower GI endoscopy. Endoscopy 2001;33(10):901–3.

81. Omori T, Kamiya Y, Tahara T, et al. Correlation between magnifying narrow band imaging and histopathology in gastric protruding/or polypoid lesions: a pilot feasibility trial. BMC Gastroenterol 2012;12:17.

82. Tanioka Y, Yanai H, Sakaguchi E. Ultraslim endoscopy with flexible spectral imaging color enhancement for upper gastrointestinal neoplasms. World J Gastrointest Endosc 2011;3(1):11–5.

83. Mouri R, Yoshida S, Tanaka S, et al. Evaluation and validation of computed virtual chromoendoscopy in early gastric cancer. Gastrointest Endosc 2009;69(6):1052–8.

84. Jung SW, Lim KS, Lim JU, et al. Flexible spectral imaging color enhancement (FICE) is useful to discriminate among non-neoplastic lesion, adenoma, and cancer of stomach. Dig Dis Sci 2011;56(10):2879–86.

85. Pasechnikov V, Chukov S, Fedorov E, et al. Gastric cancer: prevention, screening and early diagnosis. World J Gastroenterol 2014;20(38):13842–62.

86. Graham DY, Schwartz JT, Cain GD, et al. Prospective evaluation of biopsy number in the diagnosis of esophageal and gastric carcinoma. Gastroenterology 1982;82(2):228–31.

87. Waddell T, Verheij M, Allum W, et al. Gastric cancer: ESMO-ESSO-ESTRO clinical practice guidelines for diagnosis, treatment and follow-up. Eur J Surg Oncol 2014;40(5):584–91.

88. Ajani JA, D'Amico TA, Almhanna K, et al. Gastric Cancer. NCCN clinical practice guidelines in Oncology (NCCN guidelines). National Comprehensive Cancer Network, Inc; 2015. Version 3.2015. Available at: https://www.nccn.org/professionals/physician_gls/PDF/gastric.pdf. Accessed February 10, 2016.

89. Kantsevoy SV, Adler DG, Conway JD, et al. Endoscopic mucosal resection and endoscopic submucosal dissection. Gastrointest Endosc 2008;68(1):11–8.

90. Kim SG. Endoscopic treatment for early gastric cancer. J Gastric Cancer 2011;11(3):146–54.

91. Chung IK, Lee JH, Lee SH, et al. Therapeutic outcomes in 1000 cases of endoscopic submucosal dissection for early gastric neoplasms: Korean ESD Study Group multicenter study. Gastrointest Endosc 2009;69(7):1228–35.

92. Park YM, Cho E, Kang HY, et al. The effectiveness and safety of endoscopic submucosal dissection compared with endoscopic mucosal resection for early gastric cancer: a systematic review and metaanalysis. Surg Endosc 2011;25(8):2666–77.

93. Blakely AM, Miner TJ. Surgical considerations in the treatment of gastric cancer. Gastroenterol Clin North Am 2013;42(2):337–57.

94. Hudis CA. Trastuzumab–mechanism of action and use in clinical practice. N Engl J Med 2007;357(1):39–51.

95. Bang YJ, Van Cutsem E, Feyereislova A, et al. Trastuzumab in combination with chemotherapy versus chemotherapy alone for treatment of HER2-positive advanced gastric or gastro-oesophageal junction cancer (ToGA): a phase 3, open-label, randomised controlled trial. Lancet 2010;376(9742):687–97.

96. Fuchs CS, Tomasek J, Yong CJ, et al. Ramucirumab monotherapy for previously treated advanced gastric or gastro-oesophageal junction adenocarcinoma (REGARD): an international, randomised, multicentre, placebo-controlled, phase 3 trial. Lancet 2014;383(9911):31–9.

97. Siegel R, Ma J, Zou Z, et al. Cancer statistics, 2014. CA Cancer J Clin 2014;64(1):9–29.

98. Crew KD, Neugut AI. Epidemiology of gastric cancer. World J Gastroenterol 2006;12(3):354–62.

99. Surveillance, Epidemiology, and End Results (SEER) Program Research Data (1973-2010), National Cancer Institute, DCCPS, Surveillance Research Program, Surveillance Systems Branch, released April 2013, based on the November 2012 submission. Available at: www.seer.cancer.gov. Accessed January 26, 2016.

100. Dassen AE, Lemmens VE, van de Poll-Franse LV, et al. Trends in incidence, treatment and survival of gastric adenocarcinoma between 1990 and 2007: a population-based study in the Netherlands. Eur J Cancer 2010;46(6):1101–10.

# Pancreatic Cancer: A Review

Cinthya S. Yabar, MD, Jordan M. Winter, MD*

## KEYWORDS

- Pancreatic cancer • Pancreatic ductal adenocarcinoma • Evaluation • Treatment

## KEY POINTS

- Pancreatic ductal adenocarcinoma cancer is the 12th most common cancer in the United States, and pancreatic cancer deaths have been increasing steadily over the past few years.
- The genetics and other molecular aspects of pancreatic cancer have been well-characterized, with recent progress toward subtyping pancreatic tumors, with potential implications for therapy.
- The greatest risk factor for pancreatic cancer is a strong family history; environmental and medical factors have been associated (tobacco use and a history of chronic pancreatitis).
- There is no established method of early detection, and pancreatic cancer is frequently diagnosed in late stages.
- Immunotherapy and targeting DNA repair deficiency in a subset of tumors are promising areas of research and may yield improved outcomes in the near future.

## INTRODUCTION AND PUBLIC HEALTH CONCERNS

Pancreatic ductal adenocarcinoma (PDA) is the 12th most common cancer in the United States. As of January 7, 2016, the American Cancer Society reported that pancreatic cancer had surpassed breast cancer as the third leading cause of cancer related death in the United States.[1] Within the next decade, annual PDA deaths will likely surpass colorectal cancer as well. There were 53,070 new cases of PDA in 2015, and 41,780 deaths in the United States alone. Although the death rates for the most common cancers have declined in recent decades, the death rate for PDA is actually flat to slightly increased, in large part related to the aging demographic.[2,3] Over the past 4 decades, disease-specific survival has only improved marginally, with 5-year survival rates increasing from 4% to 7%. The lack of clinical progress, in comparison with other cancers, is attributable to a failure to develop novel and effective therapies. Standard treatment still consists of relatively old cytotoxic therapies. The only advance has been improved experience and success administering

Potential/Real Conflicts of Interest: None.
Department of Surgery, Thomas Jefferson University Hospital, Sidney Kimmel Medical College, 1015 Walnut Street, Curtis Building, Suite 620, Philadelphia, PA 19107, USA
* Corresponding author.
E-mail address: Jordan.Winter@jefferson.edu

combinations of drugs, which confer a small survival advantage over single agent therapy.[4–8] Mutation targeted and immunologic therapies that have shown efficacy or promise for other cancer types have not yet achieved comparable benefits for pancreatic cancer.[7–13] Herein, we review the molecular and clinical aspects of pancreatic cancer, and highlight the most critical challenges facing the management of this disease.

## MOLECULAR PATHWAYS/GENETICS

Unlike other common cancers, there are currently no well-established and evidence based treatment strategies based on molecular profiling for PDA. Similarly, there are no molecular signatures to improve staging or prognostication. However, numerous studies have been performed that have elucidated common genetic abnormalities in PDA, which highlight potential molecular targets and reveal signaling pathways that are important for disease development.[14,15] Whole-exome sequencing was performed in 24 PDA genomes, and more than 1300 different genes were mutated in these tumors.[14] The only high-frequency, "actionable" oncogene was KRAS, which is genetically activated in more than 95% of PDAs. Unfortunately, targeted therapy against this gene has proved elusive.[16] In light of this disappointing finding, various alternative approaches to personalized therapy have been proposed. Jones and colleagues[14] have grouped the common genetic abnormalities in PDA into 12 core signaling pathways (eg, apoptosis, DNA damage, and others), with the hope that biologic pathways may be more modifiable than specific gene targets. Biankin and colleagues[15] identified axon guidance genes as a novel molecular pathway with frequent gene mutations in PDA. Perhaps most compelling, there is evidence that a high proportion PDAs harbor functional defects in DNA damage pathways (approximately 25%), which may render these tumors more susceptible to certain agents that target the DNA repair process.[17] Many of the genes are Fanconi anemia pathway genes (BRCA2, PALB2, FANCC, FANCG), and clinical and preclinical data suggest that affected tumors are particularly sensitive to poly adenosine diphosphate ribose polymerase inhibitors or platinum drugs. Although phase II and III trials examining poly adenosine diphosphate ribose polymerase inhibitors in PDA are ongoing, completed studies in other cancer types (eg, ovarian) give hope that a personalized treatment approach is on the horizon (**Table 1**).[18]

Oncogenic KRAS remains the best characterized oncogene in PDA. The genetic event occurs early in tumorigenesis, before the development of invasive disease. Activated KRAS activates multiple signaling pathways including BRAF/MAP-K to affect cell proliferation, PI3K/mammalian target of rapamycin to promote cell growth and survival, and phospholipase C/PKC/Ca$^{++}$ to induce calcium and second messenger signaling.[19] KRAS mutations form the foundation of the most commonly used transgenic mouse model of PDA.[20] The mutation is combined typically with an abnormal tumor suppressor gene in these models, such as TP53.

Other high-frequency mutation genes are classified as tumor suppressor genes (CDKN2A, TP53, and SMAD4). These genes are often inactivated through a mutation in 1 allele, combined with genetic loss (ie, loss of heterozygosity) in the corresponding chromosome region of the second allele as a result of chromosomal instability. Areas where genetic loss most frequently occurs are nonrandom in the PDA genome, because they typically occur at loci containing the abovementioned tumor suppressor genes: CDKN2A (9p), TP53 (19p), and SMAD4 (18q). The most common gene mutations in PDA are provided in **Table 2**.[14,15]

**Table 1**
**Notable current PARP inhibitor trials**

| Cancer Type | Phase | Study Description (Sponsor) | Status |
|---|---|---|---|
| Ovarian | II | Olaparib as maintenance therapy for relapsed platinum-sensitive ovarian cancer (AstraZeneca) | Complete |
| | II, III | Cediranib and olaparib vs cediranib or olaparib alone, or standard of care chemotherapy in recurrent platinum-resistant or -refractory cancer; randomized (NCI) | Ongoing |
| | III | Maintenance with niraparib vs placebo in platinum sensitive cancer; randomized (Tesaro) | Ongoing |
| | III | Carboplatin/paclitaxel ± concurrent and continuation maintenance veliparib in previously untreated stages III or IV high-grade serous epithelial tumors (AbbVie) | Ongoing |
| Breast | III | Carboplatin and paclitaxel ± Veliparib in HER2-negative unresectable BRCA-associated breast cancer; randomized (AbbVie) | Ongoing |
| | III | Talazoparib in advanced, BRCA mutant cancer; randomized, 2-arm (Medivation, NBCC) | Ongoing |
| | III | Olaparib monotherapy vs chemotherapy in metastatic cancer with germline BRCA1/2 mutations; randomized (AstraZeneca) | Ongoing |
| | III | Gemcitabine/carboplatin, ± BSI-201 in ER-, PR-, and Her2-negative metastatic cancer; randomized (Sanofi) | Complete |
| | III | Niraparib vs physician's choice in HER2 negative, germline BRCA mutation cancer; randomized (Tesaro, EORTC) | Ongoing |
| Pancreas | I | PARP inhibitor in combination with gemcitabine (AstraZeneca) | Complete |
| | I, II | ABT-888 with modified FOLFOX6 in metastases; single arm (Georgetown University, Abbott) | Ongoing |
| | II | Gemcitabine and cisplatin ± veliparib or veliparib alone; randomized (NCI) | Ongoing |
| | II | Rucaparib in BRCA-mutant cancer; single arm (Clovis) | Ongoing |
| | III | Maintenance olaparib monotherapy in gBRCA mutant cancer; randomized (AstraZeneca) | Ongoing |

*Abbreviations:* EORTC, European Organization for Research and Treatment of Cancer; ER, estrogen receptor; NBCC, National Breast Cancer Coalition; NCI, National Cancer Institute; PARP, poly adenosine diphosphate ribose polymerase; PR, progesterone receptor.

*Data from* ClinicalTrials.gov. Bethesda (MD): National Library of Medicine; National Institute of Health; 2016. Available at: http://clinicaltrials.gov. Accessed April 13, 2016.

Pathologic and genetic studies reveal that PDA develops over many years, and follows an adenoma-to-carcinoma sequence, as has been described for other cancer types. Histologic atypia progresses over time through pancreatic intraepithelial neoplasia (PanIN) stages (1–3), and ultimately into invasive disease.[21] In the tumorigenesis timeline, KRAS activation and telomere shortening are among the first events to occur in tumorigenesis, followed by p16 loss in the PanIN-2 stage, and TP53, SMAD4, and BRCA2 inactivation in the PanIN-3 stage. E-cadherin loss is a late event, and leads to epithelial-to-mesenchymal transition and a highly lethal phenotype in very advanced stages.[22] Recent molecular analyses of pancreatic precursor lesions and PDA have determined that this process occurs over 10 to 20 years.[23]

Genetic sequencing studies reveal significant intratumoral heterogeneity in PDA with respect to genetic abnormalities. For instance, Iacobuzio-Donahue and

**Table 2**
**Significantly mutated pathways in pancreatic ductal adenocarcinoma**

| Core Pathway | Gene | Protein Function | Mutation Rate (%)[a] |
|---|---|---|---|
| KRAS signaling | KRAS | Oncogene; GTPase; activates MARK activity | 100 |
| | MAP2K4 | Dual specificity mitogen-activated protein kinase 4; Toll-like receptor signaling pathway | |
| DNA damage control | TP53 | Tumor suppressor p53 | 83 |
| Control of G1/S phase transition | CDKN2A | Cyclin-dependent kinase inhibitor 2A; tumor suppressor | 83–96 |
| TGF-β signaling | SMAD4 | Mothers against decapentaplegic homolog 4; BMP signaling pathway | 63–100 |
| | TGFBR2 | TGF-β receptor type II; regulation of growth | |

Abbreviations: BMP, bone morphogenetic protein; TGF, transforming growth factor.
[a] Depending on which gene expressed in sample of tumor studied.
Data from Jones S, Zhang X, Parsons DW, et al. Core signaling pathways in human pancreatic cancers revealed by global genomic analyses. Science 2008;321:1801–6; and Biankin AV, Waddell N, Kassahn KS, et al. Pancreatic cancer genomes reveal aberrations in axon guidance pathway genes. Nature 2012;491:399–405.

colleagues[24] demonstrated that founder mutations (mutations that arise early in tumorigenesis) are present throughout a tumor, yet progressor mutations (found in subclonal population of cells) are typically present in geospatial niches in the primary tumor and only in a subset of metastatic deposits. This has implications for therapy: targeted therapies designed against progressor mutations may only affect a subset of cancer clones.

Although most genetic mutations in PDA are somatic, germline variants have been described that predispose individuals to the development of PDA. Overall, 10% of PDAs are familial, and only 10% of those have been assigned to a previously defined genetic syndrome. Hereditary breast and ovarian cancer is the most common familial syndrome, and Peutz-Jeghers syndrome holds the greatest lifetime risk for the development of pancreatic cancer (approximately 30%). Other familial disorders linked to PDA include familial atypical multiple-mole melanoma and hereditary nonpolyposis colorectal cancer.[25] Many of the familial syndromes are secondary to germline mutations in the Fanconi anemia DNA repair pathway or alternative DNA repair genes, like ATM, BRCA2, FANCC, FANCG, and PALB2.

Aside from genetic abnormalities, other molecular changes have also been shown to be critical in PDA development, such as epigenetic abnormalities (methylation and histone modification), transcriptional regulation, and posttranscriptional regulation (microRNAs and RNA-binding proteins).[26]

## RISK FACTORS

PDA is most often seen in the elderly population, because it results from acquired genetic defects over many years.[23] The median age of onset is 71 years, and 75% of patients are diagnosed between the ages of 55 and 84 years.[2] The age-adjusted incidence rate is 12 out of 100,00 in the United States, and the lifetime risk of developing PDA is 1.5%, or 1 in 67 people. Of note, African Americans have a slightly increased risk compared with Caucasians.[2]

The greatest risk factor for developing PDA is having a strong family history. As mentioned, 10% to 15% of all pancreatic cancers are considered familial, which is defined as at least 2 affected first-degree relatives (FDRs, eg, parents, offspring, siblings).[27] The lifetime risk for patients with 3 or more FDRs is 40%, 10% for 2 FDRs, and 6% for 1 FDR (a 4.6-fold increase compared with the general population).[28]

In addition to genetic risk factors, the Pancreatic Cancer Case Control Consortium (PanC4, http://panc4.org/index.html) has evaluated many environmental risk factors through rigorous metaanalyses. Smoking is the best characterized and validated environmental risk factor for PDA. Active smokers have an increased relative risk of 1.74,[29] and the number of daily cigarettes directly correlates to the risk of developing PDA. Interestingly, cigars are associated with an increased risk, whereas smokeless tobacco is not.[30] Individuals with a family history and who smoke carry twice the risk compared with those high-risk patients who do not smoke.[31,32] The risk of developing PDA decreases in former smokers, and has the potential to return to baseline after 20 years of smoking cessation. Other risk factors are described in **Table 3**.[33–40] Enhanced risk associated with recent pancreatitis or diabetes (compared with chronic disease) is most likely attributable to the respective diagnoses doubling as presenting symptoms of PDA, as opposed to true causal risk factors.

## EARLY DETECTION

There are no validated early detection strategies for PDA, even for high-risk patients. Nevertheless, options are available and have been reported. Whole-body computed tomography (CT) screening for healthy patients has been described, and is offered commercially at selected imaging centers, yet data are lacking to support usefulness

**Table 3**
**Risk factors associated with pancreatic ductal adenocarcinoma**

| Risk Factor | Odds Ratio |
| --- | --- |
| Genetics | |
| >1 FDR | 4.26[33] |
| 1 FDR | 1.76[33] |
| Environmental | |
| Smoking | 1.74 |
| Chlorinated hydrocarbons | 1.4–4.1[34] |
| Polycyclic aromatic hydrocarbons | 1.1–1.5[34] |
| Heavy consumption (>8 drinks/d) | 1.6[35] |
| Medical | |
| Chronic pancreatitis | |
| >2 y of disease | 2.7 |
| <2 y of disease[a] | 13.6[36] |
| Obesity | 1–1.5[37] |
| Diabetes mellitus, type II | |
| Long-standing disease | 1.4–1.8[38] |
| Recent onset (<2 y)[a] | 2.9[39,40] |

*Abbreviation:* FDR, first-degree relative.
[a] Likely represent presenting symptomatology as opposed to causal factor.

of this practice for routine cancer screening. Downsides include high cost, radiation exposure, and an high incidence of false-positive or low-consequence findings.[41] High-risk populations, such as individuals with a family history, may benefit from surveillance using endoscopic ultrasonography, CT, or MRI.[42] The Cancer of the Pancreas Screening Project (CAPS study) is an ongoing prospective study to better evaluate screening strategies in such high-risk patients. Unfortunately, available data indicate that the sensitivity of screening programs even in high-risk groups remains low, and the most commonly identified lesions are cysts, as opposed to conventional PDA.[43] Recently, a 49-member multidisciplinary panel at the International CAPS Consortium summit generated screening recommendations for high-risk patients best on available data and expert opinion. Screening by endoscopic ultrasonography and MRI is recommended for patients with at least 2 FDRs, Peutz-Jeghers syndrome, hereditary nonpolyposis colon cancer mutation with 1 FDR, or individuals with germline mutations in p16 (*CDKN2A*) or *BRCA2*. Surveillance should be performed annually and begin around 50 years of age. Any suspicious mass should be further evaluated by CT. Among their recommendations, the panel also made a point to discuss the possibility and potential dangers of false positives and the implications of these findings.[44]

Conceptually speaking, early detection remains a holy grail for PDA management. Patients who present with "early" disease in fact typically have occult micrometastatic disease that becomes clinically relevant within the first 2 years after resection.[45] A recent study of small invasive intraductal papillary mucinous neoplasms (<2 cm invasive component) reveals that a large proportion of small or early PDAs recur after resection, even in the absence of lymph node metastases.[46] Moreover, owing to limitations in modern imaging, conventional PDA (not associated with a cystic component) rarely presents at the T1 or even T2 stage.[47,48] Ideally, PDA would be detected and treated at the PanIN 3 stage (carcinoma in situ); this would maximize cures and at the same time minimize any unnecessary treatment or overtreatment that would inevitably follow treatment of earlier PanIN lesions. Autopsy studies reveal that the incidence of PanIN 3 is similar to PDA, suggesting that most of these premalignant cases progress to PDA in patients' lifetimes.[49] Yachida and colleagues[23] measured passenger mutations in PDAs, and determined mathematically that the disease develops over roughly 20 years. These data provide a glimmer of hope that early detection remains a possibility.

Current technologies, however, offer little promise for successful early detection, using PanIN 3 as the desired target lesion. PDA is difficult to image with present-day capabilities. Pancreatic masses are difficult to appreciate, and often are only implied based on the appearance of dilated or obstructed ducts, or atrophic pancreata (all findings consistent with long-standing disease). Indeed, invasive lesions (let alone PanIN 3) are rarely apparent when they are less than 2 cm.[46] It must be emphasized that an effective screening test for PDA, with applicability for the general population, must be extraordinarily accurate owing to low disease prevalence. A test with 99% accuracy would still result in a 1% false-positive rate, which is unacceptably high,[50] because treatment of suspected lesions requires an invasive operation. Moreover, this rate actually approaches the mortality rate of pancreatectomy in high-volume centers. There are significant efforts to determine if blood-based analytes (ie, liquid biopsies) can be used as a minimally invasive and inexpensive screening option. For example, investigators at the M.D. Anderson Cancer Center recently published an analysis of exosomes in the serum, which can protect circulating nucleic acids and, therefore, may be informative.[51] This line of research, however, is somewhat fraught with unfulfilled promise, because circulating markers of PDA are likely evidence that the disease is already beyond curable. Successful studies of liquid biopsies often show that that the test can detect PDA that is already clinically evident and, therefore, do not show any advantage over standard diagnostic strategies (like CT and serum CA 19–9). Thus, this line of research is better suited to measure burden of disease and response to therapy in patients with clinically measurable disease, as opposed to early, premalignant and curable disease.

## DIAGNOSTIC EVALUATION

Evaluation of the patient with pancreatic cancer involves a detailed history and physical examination, laboratory tests, and appropriate imaging. The patient history should include questions about risk factors for pancreatic cancer and common pre-senting symptoms. The initial presentation of a patient is related to the location of the tumor. In patients with a mass in the right side of the pancreas (ie, head, neck, or uncinate process), jaundice (75%) often occurs from obstruction of the common bile duct; other symptoms include weight loss (50%), abdominal pain (40%), new-onset diabetes (10%), and nausea (10%). Pancreatic duct obstruction is often associated with acute pancreatitis and steatorrhea from exocrine insuffi-ciency. Left-sided lesions (the body or tail) frequently present with abdominal pain, back pain, diabetes, or nausea. Laboratory testing should include a complete blood count (principally to evaluate for anemia) and a complete metabolic panel (to evaluate for abnormal liver transaminases and function). A coagulation profile should be drawn, because biliary obstruction can lead to vitamin K deficiency. The physical examination should be focused on key findings such as scleral icterus, jaundice, and lymphadenopathy.

Cross-sectional imaging evaluation is necessary for a pancreatic or periampullary mass and proper staging of the patient. Additional evaluation and treatment recom-mendations are contingent on the perceived stage (1 and 2 is resectable or border-line, 3 is locally advanced, and 4 is metastatic, **Table 4** provides the American Joint Committee on Cancer TNM staging schema for exocrine pancreatic cancer).[52] The preferred imaging modality is a triphasic CT scan, with an early arterial phase, late arterial phase (parenchymal), and portal venous phase. The study is performed with thin slices (2.5–5 mm), 3-dimensional reconstruction, and uses water as an oral contrast agent.[53] Chest imaging (radiograph or CT) is performed in search for pul-monary metastases. PET/CT imaging adds little additional value beyond these studies. Endoscopic ultrasonography is performed for unresectable disease to obtain a definitive tissue-based diagnosis before chemotherapy. The test is not necessary for many resectable lesions when a high degree of suspicion for PDA is present because these individuals are managed with resection; however, the test has value in selected cases where alternative diagnoses are likely (eg, pancreatitis).

## CLINICAL MANAGEMENT

Management of the patient with PDA is based on the extent of disease. Patients with local disease (stages I and II) are evaluated for resection, and offered surgical therapy if they are considered medically fit for pancreatectomy, and the tumor is considered resectable based on available imaging studies (eg, CT). General guidelines of resect-ability follow 'surgical' staging criteria, which generally overlap with TNM staging, but are designed specifically with surgical anatomy in mind.[54] Thus, these criteria focus on the involvement of the major visceral vessels in the upper abdomen (portal vein, supe-rior mesenteric vein, superior mesenteric artery, hepatic artery, and celiac artery).

| Table 4 | |
|---|---|
| **TNM pancreatic cancer staging system** | |
| T categories | |
| Tis | Carcinoma in situ |
| T1 | Mass ≤2 cm, confined to the pancreas |
| T2 | Mass >2 cm, still confined to the pancreas |
| T3 | Mass that extends beyond the pancreas |
| T4 | Mass invades visceral arteries (ie, locally advanced) |
| N categories | |
| N0 | No affected lymph nodes |
| N1 | Regional lymph node metastases |
| M categories | |
| M0 | No evidence of metastases |
| M1 | Distant metastases |
| Stage grouping for pancreatic cancer[a] | |
| Stage 0 | Tis, N0, M0 |
| Stage IA | T1, N0, M0 |
| Stage IB | T2, N0, M0 |
| Stage IIA | T3, N0, M0 |
| Stage IIB | T1-3, N1, M0 |
| Stage III | T4, any N, M0 |
| Stage IV | Any T, any N, M1 |

[a] Information from the American Joint Committee on Cancer 7th edition TNM staging system.[51]
Used with permission of the American Joint Committee on Cancer (AJCC), Chicago, Illinois. The original and primary source for this information is the AJCC Cancer Staging Manual, Seventh Edition (2010) published by Springer Science+Business Media.

Localized PDAs are categorized as resectable, borderline resectable, or locally advanced, and generally reflect the likelihood of obtaining a complete resection (R0 for resectable, R1 for borderline, and R2 for locally advanced; see **Fig. 1**). The accompanying **Table 5** provides generally accepted definitions for these categories.[55] Resectable and borderline resectable PDAs are typically stage II cancers; locally advanced disease is tantamount to stage II. Patients with locally advanced disease are typically offered chemotherapy, and sometimes chemoradiation, as a neoadjuvant treatment approach, with a goal of reducing disease burden and perhaps with an eye toward resection in the future in a minority of cases (10%).[56] Patients with borderline resectable disease are offered neoadjuvant therapy frequently (chemotherapy, chemoradiation, or both), with a greater percentage eventually undergoing a resection (60%).[57] Opinions vary on the sequence of treatment for resectable PDA (surgery or neoadjuvant treatment first), and randomized trials have not been conducted to address this specific question. Patients with stage IV disease are offered systemic chemotherapy when they have an appropriate performance status to suggest they will tolerate such treatment.

In addition to a tissue diagnosis, patients undergoing nonoperative management often require palliation to relieve biliary or duodenal obstruction if present. This can usually be achieved endoscopically, although percutaneous approaches are also options. Self-expanding metallic stents are now used routinely by therapeutic endoscopists to manage jaundice, and effectively decompress the biliary system for several

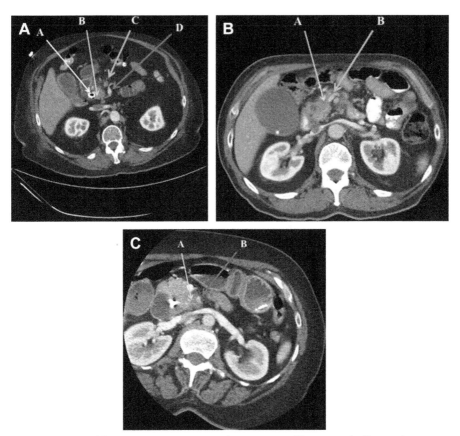

**Fig. 1.** (*A*) Resectable pancreatic cancer. A indicates a metallic stent; B indicates the pancreatic adenocarcinoma; C indicates a free superior mesenteric vein; D indicates a free superior mesenteric artery. (*B*) Borderline resectable pancreatic cancer. A indicates the adenocarcinoma; B indicates an encased and distorted superior mesenteric vein. (*C*) Unresectable pancreatic cancer. A indicates the adenocarcinoma; B indicates an encased and distorted superior mesenteric artery.

months. Regardless of the stage or approach, a multidisciplinary team is important to address the oncologic, psychological, nutritional, and somatic aspects of PDA.

## SURGERY

As stated, resectional therapy is offered to many patients with localized disease. Pancreaticoduodenectomy (PD) is performed for right-sided pancreatic cancers, where the specimen includes gallbladder, duodenum, head of pancreas, proximal jejunum, and distal common bile duct. Gastrointestinal reconstruction is required to restore intestinal continuity, and includes pancreaticojejunostomy, hepaticojejunostomy, and enteroenterostomy (duodenojejunostomy for a pylorus preserving resection or gastrojejunostomy when the pylorus is resected). Distal pancreatectomy is performed for cancers of the body or tail with an en bloc splenectomy for a more comprehensive lymphadenectomy. Minimally invasive approaches have been used and reported, with comparable outcomes to the open approach in high-volume centers.[58]

**Table 5**
**Guidelines of surgical staging criteria[a]**

| Clinical Stage | American Joint Committee on Cancer Stage | Relationship to Major Vessel on CT Imaging | | | |
|---|---|---|---|---|---|
| | | Superior Mesenteric Artery | Celiac Axis | Common Hepatic Artery | Superior Mesenteric Vein-Portal Vein Confluence |
| Resectable | I/II | Normal tissue plane | Normal tissue plane | Normal tissue plane | Patent, but tumor may be abutting or encasing vessel. The vein is reconstructable. |
| Borderline resectable | II or III | Abutment | Abutment | Abutment, or short segment encasement[b] | May have short segment occlusion, but reconstruction is possible. |
| Locally advanced | III | Encasement | Encasement | Extensive encasement with no technical option for reconstruction | Occlusion with no technical option for resection or reconstruction. |

[a] Based on the Varadhachary/Katz CT staging system for adenocarcinoma of the pancreatic head and uncinate process.[55]
[b] Defined as greater than 180° of vessel encasement.
*Data from* Katz MH, Pisters PW, Evans DB, et al. Borderline resectable pancreatic cancer: the importance of this emerging stage of disease. J Am Coll Surg 2008;206(5):833–46.

Mortality rates after PD has improved significantly in recent decades and is less than 5% at high-volume centers.[43] However, morbidity after PD remains high (40%). The most common complications after PD include pancreatic leak (20%), delayed gastric emptying (15%), and wound infection (10%).[45] The International Study Group of Pancreatic Surgery works to standardize definitions and criteria for pancreatic surgery-related complications and results to enhance the use of reported outcomes. This consortium has provided guidelines and definitions for pancreatic leaks,[59] delayed gastric emptying,[60] and hemorrhage,[61] in addition to establishing strict guidelines for reporting aspects related to the pancreatic remnant and anastomosis.[62] For instance, duct size, gland texture, mobilization distance, type of anastomosis, suture used, and use of stent are some characteristics requiring reporting to better standardize both the procedural terms and outcome evaluation.[62]

## CHEMOTHERAPY

Fifty percent of patients diagnosed with PDA are diagnosed with metastatic disease at presentation.[3] Chemotherapy is palliative in this setting, and the principal goals are to control disease and improve quality of life.

To monitor for toxicities, patients undergo weekly laboratory testing, and are seen biweekly or monthly by their medical oncologist. Treatment responses are monitored by CT scans every 8 weeks, as well as serum carbohydrate antigen (CA)19-9 levels at the same interval. If the patient does not express CA19-9 owing to a Lewis antigen polymorphism (10% of patients), carcinoembryonic antigen or CA-125 can be serially followed.[63]

## SURVIVORSHIP

There are no robust predictors of favorable cancer-specific survival in patients with PDA. For patients undergoing resection, conventional pathologic features are the most informative for this purpose, and adverse factors include lymph node metastasis, poor differentiation, tumor size greater than 3 cm, and positive resection margins.[47] However, these individual factors have weak prognostic value, with multivariate Cox proportional hazard ratios around only 1.5.[47] In other words, adverse pathologic features do not preclude long survival, and favorable features do not exclude the possibility of early recurrence and death after resection. For example, lymph node metastases are absent in roughly 20% of short-term survivors (<12 months).[64]

Aside from pathologic features, the most informative and routinely used prognostic marker in patients undergoing resection is the postoperative CA19-9 level. In the best scenarios, CA19-9 returns to normal levels by 1 month after resection. As shown in the landmark Radiation Therapy Oncology Group 9704 adjuvant trial, levels greater than 180 U/mL are associated with a multivariate proportional hazard ratio of 3.6.[63] However, CA19-9 is not expressed in roughly 10% of patients' tumors, and therefore will not be informative in these cases. Interestingly, patients with tumors that do not express CA19-9 may actually have improved survival, for unknown reasons.

According to National Comprehensive Cancer Network guidelines, patients undergoing resection should undergo surveillance every 3 to 6 months for 2 years, then annually thereafter for patients who have had a mass resected. A history and physical examination, surveillance CT scans of the chest and abdomen with oral and intravenous contrast, and trending tumor markers are recommended for a complete assessment. The median survival after resection for PDA remains about 18 months in large institutional series.[45] Unfortunately, improvement in cancer-specific survival in patients undergoing resection has not improved over the past 30 years.[65] On average, patients recur roughly 1 year after resection.[66] Overall survival is typically longer (approximately 20–22 months) in randomized adjuvant trials, where favorable patient selection for the trial occurs.[67,68] These cohorts exclude patients who have a prolonged recovery from surgery, opt against adjuvant therapy, or experience early recurrences. Recurrences typically occur in the retroperitoneum (57%), liver (51%), peritoneum (35%), and lung (15%). The most common pattern of failure includes recurrences at both distant and local sites (46%), followed by metastatic sites only (33%), and local recurrence only (12%).[69]

Patients with stage III disease have an average overall survival of 12 months.[70] There is some evidence that patients with SMAD4-positive tumors have a local predominant progression pattern, whereas tumors with absent SMAD4 expression have a disseminated pattern of failure.[24,70] If validated, this biomarker can be used to select patients having locally advanced disease for intensified local therapy (eg, radiation), as well as patients who would likely not benefit from such an approach. Current trials are ongoing to explore this treatment strategy (NCT01921751, NCT02241551).[18] Although SMAD4 may be predictive of recurrence pattern for patients with stage III disease, the biomarker seems to be less informative in resected specimens.[69] Median overall survival for patients with stage IV disease is less than 6 months, but in recent prospective randomized trials, survival approaches 1 year for patients with the highest performance status, and who receive multiagent chemotherapeutic regimens (eg, FOLFIRINOX).[5,71,72]

## FUTURE DIRECTIONS

Other cancer types have benefited from substantial advances in experimental therapeutic research, which include the development of small molecule and antibody targeted therapies, as well as novel immunologic therapies. For instance, patients with HER2-positive breast cancer or BRAF mutant melanoma experience a survival advantage that can exceed 1 year with mutation targeted therapies.[73,74] Immunologic checkpoint inhibitors achieve similar survival benefits for patients with melanoma.[75,76] Although investigators have attempted to repurpose these molecular therapeutic strategies for PDA, their effect seems to be far less robust. There were no responders to an anti–PD-L1 inhibitor with PDA.[11] Epidermal growth factor receptor inhibition with erlotinib produced just a 10-day survival benefit in patients with metastatic PDA.[77] In contrast with colon cancer, wild-type KRAS did not predict response.[78] Similarly, targeting HER2 has not been effective to treat HER2-positive PDA.[79] Although KRAS is mutated in more than 90% of PDAs, attempts to target this oncogene have also failed.[16] Therefore, it is likely that significant advances will require innovative, disease-specific strategies. For instance, efforts are ongoing to target the tenacious stromal reaction within PDA to facilitate drug delivery. A promising approach is to degrade hyaluronic acid enzymatically using recombinant human hyaluronidase,[80] which is being examined in a current clinical trial together with combination chemotherapy in metastatic pancreatic cancer patients (NCT01959139).[18] Scientists continue to explore ways to encourage immunologic responses to PDA, by combining check point inhibitors and other immunologic agents. Further investigations into the molecular mechanisms that drive PDA survival and adaptation to severe metabolic conditions in the tumor microenvironment may uncover novel therapeutic targets with a sufficient therapeutic window.[81] Perhaps the line of research with the quickest payoff is a personalized therapeutic approach using poly adenosine diphosphate ribose polymerase inhibitors to treat PDAs that have genetic deficiencies in DNA repair mechanisms (eg, BRCA2, PALB2, FANCC, FANCG).[17] Clinical trials are underway to study this approach, which may have relevance to as many as 25% of patients with PDA (NCT00515866, NCT02042378, NCT02498613, NCT01585805, NCT00047307, NCT02184195, NCT01489865, NCT01286987, NCT00576654, NCT00892736, NCT01989546, and NCT01078662).[18]

## SUMMARY

As the third leading cause of cancer-related death in the United States, PDA is truly a public health problem, and underfunded at that. There has been some progress toward understanding the disease at a molecular level, but genetic and other molecular advances have had a minimal impact on improving outcomes for patients. Surgery can be performed safely in appropriately selected patients, but most patients recur after resection, and the majority of patients with PDA present with advanced disease and are not candidates for resection. Clinical progress in the management of advanced disease has been limited to multiagent chemotherapy regimens that offer a relatively short survival advantage, at the price of added cost and significant toxicity. There is an urgent need for innovative research that leads improves detection capabilities and to novel drugs with improved efficacy and reduced toxicity.

## REFERENCES

1. American Cancer Society. Cancer facts and figures 2016. Atlanta (GA): American Cancer Society; 2016.
2. National Cancer Institute. SEER stat fact sheets: pancreas cancer. Available at: http://seer.cancer.gov/statfacts/html/pancreas.html. Accessed January 5, 2016.
3. Siegel RL, Miller KD, Jemal A. Cancer statistics, 2016. CA Cancer J Clin 2016; 66(1):7–30.
4. Burris HA 3rd, Moore MJ, Andersen J, et al. Improvements in survival and clinical benefit with gemcitabine as first-line therapy for patients with advanced pancreas cancer: a randomized trial. J Clin Oncol 1997;15:2403–13.
5. Conroy T, Desseigne F, Ychou M, et al. FOLFIRINOX versus gemcitabine for metastatic pancreatic cancer. N Engl J Med 2011;364:1817–25.
6. Conroy T, Paillot B, Francois E, et al. Irinotecan plus oxaliplatin and leucovorin-modulated uorouracil in advanced pancreatic cancer—a Groupe Tumeurs Digestives of the Federation Nationale des Centres de Lutte Contre le Cancer study. J Clin Oncol 2005;23:1228–36.
7. Von Hoff DD, Ramanathan RK, Borad MJ, et al. Gemcitabine plus nab-paclitaxel is an active regimen in patients with advanced pancreatic cancer: a phase I/II trial. J Clin Oncol 2011;29:4548–54.
8. Von Hoff DD, Ervin T, Arena FP, et al. Increased survival in pancreatic cancer with nab-paclitaxel plus gemcitabine. N Engl J Med 2013;369:1691–703.
9. Slamon DJ, Leyland-Jones B, Shak S, et al. Use of chemotherapy plus a monoclonal antibody against HER2 for metastatic breast cancer that overexpresses HER2. N Engl J Med 2001;344:783–92.
10. Maemondo M, Inoue A, Kobayashi K, et al. Gefitinib or chemotherapy for non-small-cell lung cancer with mutated EGFR. N Engl J Med 2010;362:2380–8.
11. Brahmer JR, Tykodi SS, Chow LQ, et al. Safety and activity of anti-PD-L1 antibody in patients with advanced cancer. N Engl J Med 2012;366:2455–65.
12. Topalian SL, Hodi FS, Brahmer JR, et al. Safety, activity, and immune correlates of anti-PD-1 antibody in cancer. N Engl J Med 2012;366:2443–54.
13. Van Cutsem E, Kohne CH, Hitre E, et al. Cetuximab and chemotherapy as initial treatment for metastatic colorectal cancer. N Engl J Med 2009;360:1408–17.

14. Jones S, Zhang X, Parsons DW, et al. Core signaling pathways in human pancreatic cancers revealed by global genomic analyses. Science 2008;321:1801–6.
15. Biankin AV, Waddell N, Kassahn KS, et al. Pancreatic cancer genomes reveal aberrations in axon guidance pathway genes. Nature 2012;491:399–405.
16. Van Cutsem E, Van de Velde H, Karasek P, et al. Phase III trial of gemcitabine plus tipifarnib compared with gemcitabine plus placebo in advanced pancreatic cancer. J Clin Oncol 2004;27:1430–8.
17. Waddell N, Pajic M, Patch AM, et al. Whole genomes redefine the mutational landscape of pancreatic cancer. Nature 2015;518:495–501. http://dx.doi.org/10.1038/nature14169.
18. ClinicalTrials.gov. Bethesda (MD): National Library of Medicine; National Institute of Health; 2016. Available at: http://clinicaltrials.gov. Accessed April 13, 2016.
19. Suda K, Tomizawa K, Mitsudomi T. Biological and clinical significance of KRAS mutations in lung cancer: an oncogenic driver that contrasts with EGFR mutation. Cancer Metastasis Rev 2010;29:49–60.
20. Hingorani SR, Wang L, Multani AS, et al. Trp53R172H and KrasG12D cooperate to promote chromosomal instability and widely metastatic pancreatic ductal adenocarcinoma in mice. Cancer Cell 2005;7:469–83.
21. Wilentz RE, Iacobuzio-Donahue CA, Argani P, et al. Loss of expression of Dpc4 in pancreatic intraepithelial neoplasia: evidence that DPC4 inactivation occurs late in neoplastic progression. Cancer Res 2000;60:2002–6.
22. Winter JM, Ting AH, Vilardell F, et al. Absence of E-cadherin expression distinguishes noncohesive from cohesive pancreatic cancer. Clin Cancer Res 2008;14:412–8.
23. Yachida S, Jones S, Bozic I, et al. Distant metastasis occurs late during the genetic evolution of pancreatic cancer. Nature 2010;467:1114–7.
24. Iacobuzio-Donahue CA, Fu B, Yachida S, et al. DPC4 gene status of the primary carcinoma correlates with patterns of failure in patients with pancreatic cancer. J Clin Oncol 2009;27:1806–13.
25. Klein AP, Hruban RH, Brune K, et al. Familial pancreatic cancer. Cancer J 2001;7:266–73.
26. Winter JM, Maitra A, Yeo CJ. Genetics and pathology of pancreatic cancer. HPB (Oxford) 2006;8:324–36.
27. Klein AP. Genetic susceptibility to pancreatic cancer. Mol Carcinog 2012;51:14–24.
28. Klein AP, Brune KA, Petersen GM, et al. Prospective risk of pancreatic cancer in familial pancreatic cancer kindreds. Cancer Res 2004;64:2634–8.
29. Iodice S, Gandini S, Maisonneuve P, et al. Tobacco and the risk of pancreatic cancer: a review and meta-analysis. Langenbecks Arch Surg 2008;393:535–45.
30. Bertuccio P, La Vecchia C, Silverman DT, et al. Cigar and pipe smoking, smokeless tobacco use and pancreatic cancer: an analysis from the International Pancreatic Cancer Case-Control Consortium (PanC4). Ann Oncol 2011;22:1420–6.
31. Silverman DT, Schiffman M, Everhart J, et al. Diabetes mellitus, other medical conditions and familial history of cancer as risk factors for pancreatic cancer. Br J Cancer 1999;80:1830–7.
32. Schenk M, Schwartz AG, O'Neal E, et al. Familial risk of pancreatic cancer. J Natl Cancer Inst 2001;93:640–4.
33. Jacobs EJ, Chanock SJ, Fuchs CS, et al. Family history of cancer and risk of pancreatic cancer: a pooled analysis from the Pancreatic Cancer Cohort Consortium (PanScan). Int J Cancer 2010;127:1421–8.

34. Andreotti G, Silverman DT. Occupational risk factors and pancreatic cancer: a review of recent findings. Mol Carcinog 2012;51:98–108.

35. Lucenteforte E, La Vecchia C, Silverman D, et al. Alcohol consumption and pancreatic cancer: a pooled analysis in the International Pancreatic Cancer Case-Control Consortium (PanC4). Ann Oncol 2012;23:374–82.

36. Duell EJ, Lucenteforte E, Olson SH, et al. Pancreatitis and pancreatic cancer risk: a pooled analysis in the International Pancreatic Cancer Case-Control Consortium (PanC4). Ann Oncol 2012;23:2964–70.

37. Bracci PM. Obesity and pancreatic cancer: overview of epidemiologic evidence and biologic mechanisms. Mol Carcinog 2012;51:53–63.

38. Li D, Tang H, Hassan MM, et al. Diabetes and risk of pancreatic cancer: a pooled analysis of three large case-control studies. Cancer Causes Control 2011;22: 189–97.

39. Huxley R, Ansary-Moghaddam A, Berrington de Gonzalez A, et al. Type-II diabetes and pancreatic cancer: a meta-analysis of 36 studies. Br J Cancer 2005; 92:2076–83.

40. Ben Q, Xu M, Ning X, et al. Diabetes mellitus and risk of pancreatic cancer: a meta-analysis of cohort studies. Eur J Cancer 2011;47:1928–37.

41. Huang B, Law MW, Khong PL. Whole-body PET/CT scanning: estimation of radiation dose and cancer risk. Radiology 2009;251:166–74.

42. Winter JM, Cameron JL, Lillemoe KD, et al. Periampullary and pancreatic incidentaloma: a single institution's experience with an increasingly common diagnosis. Ann Surg 2006;243:673–80 [discussion: 680-73].

43. Canto MI, Hruban RH, Fishman EK, et al. Frequent detection of pancreatic lesions in asymptomatic high-risk individuals. Gastroenterology 2012;142:796–804.

44. Canto MI, Harinck F, Hruban RH, et al. International Cancer of the Pancreas Screening (CAPS) Consortium summit on the management of patients with increased risk for familial pancreatic cancer. Gut 2013;62:339–47.

45. Winter JM, Cameron JL, Campbell KA, et al. 1423 pancreaticoduodenectomies for pancreatic cancer: A single-institution experience. J Gastrointest Surg 2006; 10:1199–210.

46. Winter JM, Jiang W, Bastruk O, et al. Recurrence and survival after resection of small intraductal papillary mucinous neoplasm-associated carcinomas ($\leq$20-mm invasive component): a multi-institutional analysis. Ann Surg 2016;263(4): 793–801.

47. House MG, Gonen M, Jarnagin WR, et al. Prognostic significance of pathologic nodal status in patients with resected pancreatic cancer. J Gastrointest Surg 2007;11(11):1549–55.

48. Fong ZV, Tan WP, Lavu H, et al. Preoperative imaging for resectable periampullary cancer: clinicopathologic implications of reported radiographic findings. J Gastrointest Surg 2013;17(6):1098–106.

49. Kozuka S, Sassa R, Taki T, et al. Relation of pancreatic duct hyperplasia to carcinoma. Cancer 1979;43(4):1418–28.

50. Pannala R, Basu A, Petersen GM, et al. New-onset diabetes: a potential clue to the early diagnosis of pancreatic cancer. Lancet Oncol 2009;10:88–95.

51. San Lucas FA, Allenson K, Bernard V, et al. Minimally invasive genomic and transcriptomic profiling of visceral cancers by next-generation sequencing of circulating exosomes. Ann Oncol 2015. http://dx.doi.org/10.1093/annonc/mdv604.

52. Edge SE, Byrd DR. AJCC cancer staging manual. New York: Springer; 2009.

53. Wolfgang CL, Corl F, Johnson PT, et al. Pancreatic surgery for the radiologist, 2011: an illustrated review of classic and newer surgical techniques for pancreatic tumor resection. AJR Am J Roentgenol 2011;197:1343–50.

54. Evans DB, Erickson BA, Ritch P. Borderline resectable pancreatic cancer: definitions and the importance of multimodality therapy. Ann Surg Oncol 2010;17: 2803–5.

55. Katz MH, Pisters PW, Evans DB, et al. Borderline resectable pancreatic cancer: the importance of this emerging stage of disease. J Am Coll Surg 2008;206: 833–46 [discussion: 846–8].

56. Crane CH, Varadhachary GR, Yordy JS, et al. Phase II trial of cetuximab, gemcitabine, and oxaliplatin followed by chemoradiation with cetuximab for locally advanced (T4) pancreatic adenocarcinoma: correlation of Smad4(Dpc4) immunostaining with pattern of disease progression. J Clin Oncol 2011;29:3037–43.

57. Katz MH, Fleming JB, Bhosale P, et al. Response of borderline resectable pancreatic cancer to neoadjuvant therapy is not reflected by radiographic indicators. Cancer 2012;118:5749–56.

58. Kendrick ML. Laparoscopic and robotic resection for pancreatic cancer. Cancer J 2012;18:571–6.

59. Bassi C, Dervenis C, Butturini G, et al. Postoperative pancreatic fistula: an international study group (ISGPF) definition. Surgery 2005;138:8–13.

60. Wente MN, Bassi C, Dervenis, et al. Delayed gastric emptying (DGE) after pancreatic surgery: a suggested definition by the International Study Group of Pancreatic Surgery (ISGPS). Surgery 2007;142:761–8.

61. Wente MN, Veit JA, Bassi C, et al. Postpancreatectomy hemorrhage (PPH): an International Study Group of Pancreatic Surgery (ISGPS) definition. Surgery 2007; 142:20–5.

62. Shukla PJ, Barreto SG, Fingerhut A, et al. Toward improving uniformity and standardization in the reporting of pancreatic anastomoses: a new classification system by the International Study Group of Pancreatic Surgery (ISGPS). Surgery 2010;147:144–53.

63. Berger AC, Garcia M Jr, Hoffman JP, et al. Postresection CA 19-9 predicts overall survival in patients with pancreatic cancer treated with adjuvant chemoradiation: a prospective validation by RTOG 9704. J Clin Oncol 2008;26:5918–22.

64. Winter JM, Tang LH, Klimstra DS, et al. A novel survival-based tissue microarray of pancreatic cancer validates MUC1 and mesothelin as biomarkers. PLoS One 2012;7:e40157.

65. Winter JM, Brennan MF, Tang LH, et al. Survival after resection of pancreatic adenocarcinoma: results from a single institution over three decades. Ann Surg Oncol 2012;19:169–75.

66. Oettle H, Post S, Neuhaus P, et al. Adjuvant chemotherapy with gemcitabine vs observation in patients undergoing curative-intent resection of pancreatic cancer: a randomized controlled trial. JAMA 2007;297:267–77.

67. Oettle H, Neuhaus P, Hochhaus A, et al. Adjuvant chemotherapy with gemcitabine and long-term outcomes among patients with resected pancreatic cancer: the CONKO-001 randomized trial. JAMA 2013;310:1473–81.

68. Regine WF, Winter KA, Abrams R, et al. Fluorouracil-based chemoradiation with either gemcitabine or uorouracil chemotherapy after resection of pancreatic adenocarcinoma: 5-year analysis of the U.S. Intergroup/RTOG 9704 phase III trial. Ann Surg Oncol 2011;18:1319–26.

69. Winter JM, Tang LH, Klimstra DS, et al. Failure patterns in resected pancreas adenocarcinoma: lack of predicted benefit to smad4 expression. Ann Surg 2013;258:331–5.
70. Cai S, Hong TS, Goldberg SI, et al. Updated long-term outcomes and prognostic factors for patients with unresectable locally advanced pancreatic cancer treated with intraoperative radiotherapy at the Massachusetts General Hospital, 1978 to 2010. Cancer 2013;119:4196–204.
71. Riall TS, Nealon WH, Goodwin JS, et al. Pancreatic cancer in the general population: Improvements in survival over the last decade. J Gastrointest Surg 2006; 10:1212–23.
72. Ychou M, Desseigne F, Guimbaud R, et al. Randomized phase II trial comparing FOLFIRINOX (5FU/leucovorin [LV], irinotecan [I] and oxaliplatin [O]) vs gemcitabine (G) as first-line treatment for metastatic pancreatic adenocarcinoma (MPA). First results of the ACCORD 11 trial. J Clin Oncol 2007;25:4516.
73. Swain SM, Baselga J, Kim SB, et al. Pertuzumab, trastuzumab, and docetaxel in HER2-positive metastatic breast cancer. N Engl J Med 2015;372:724–34.
74. Robert C, Karaszewska B, Schachter J, et al. Improved overall survival in melanoma with combined dabrafenib and trametinib. N Engl J Med 2015;372:30–9.
75. Hamid O, Robert C, Daud A, et al. Safety and tumor responses with lambrolizumab (anti-PD-1) in melanoma. N Engl J Med 2013;369:134–44.
76. Robert C, Schachter J, Long GV, et al. Pembrolizumab versus Ipilimumab in Advanced Melanoma. N Engl J Med 2015;372:2521–32.
77. Moore MJ, Goldstein D, Hamm J, et al. Erlotinib plus gemcitabine compared with gemcitabine alone in patients with advanced pancreatic cancer: a phase III trial of the National Cancer Institute of Canada Clinical Trials Group. J Clin Oncol 2007;25:1960–6.
78. da Cunha Santos G, Dhani N, Tu D, et al. Molecular predictors of outcome in a phase 3 study of gemcitabine and erlotinib therapy in patients with advanced pancreatic cancer: National Cancer Institute of Canada Clinical Trials Group Study PA.3. Cancer 2010;116:5599–607.
79. Harder J, Ihorst G, Heinemann V, et al. Multicentre phase II trial of trastuzumab and capecitabine in patients with HER2 overexpressing metastatic pancreatic cancer. Br J Cancer 2012;106:1033–8.
80. Provenzano PP, Cuevas C, Chang AE, et al. Enzymatic targeting of the stroma ablates physical barriers to treatment of pancreatic ductal adenocarcinoma. Cancer Cell 2012;21:418–29.
81. Burkhart RA, Pineda DM, Chand SN, et al. HuR is a post-transcriptional regulator of core metabolic enzymes in pancreatic cancer. RNA Biol 2013;10:1312–23.

# Small Bowel Adenocarcinoma

Thomas Aparicio, MD, PhD[a],*, Aziz Zaanan, MD, PhD[b], Florence Mary, MD[a],
Pauline Afchain, MD[c], Sylvain Manfredi, MD, PhD[d],
Thomas Ronald Jeffry Evans, MB BS, MD, FRCP[e]

## KEYWORDS

- Rare tumor • Small intestine adenocarcinoma • Carcinogenesis • Lynch syndrome
- Prognostic factor • Chemotherapy

## KEY POINTS

- The most frequent location of small bowel adenocarcinoma is duodenum.
- Small bowel adenocarcinoma occurs in around 20% in a context of predisposing disease.
- Small bowel adenocarcinoma molecular phenotype is close to that of colorectal adenocarcinoma.
- After an R0 resection, lymph node invasion is the main prognostic factor.
- The benefit of adjuvant chemotherapy should be demonstrated by a prospective clinical trial.

## INTRODUCTION

Small bowel adenocarcinoma (SBA) is a rare cancer, but there is a growing impetus to perform multicenter or collaborative studies to answer key questions in patient management.[1] Large biological studies are now possible to potentially exploit the molecular and cellular basis of SBA development and progression to develop novel therapies. Collaboration through the International Rare Cancer Initiative has led to

BALLAD - A global study to evaluate the potential benefit of adjuvant chemotherapy for small bowel adenocarcinoma (International Rare Cancers Initiative study - IRCI 002) is supported by Cancer Research UK (Grant Award - A15828) and by Programme Hospitalier de Recherche Clinique and INCa (Grant Award – PHRC-K13-073).

[a] Gastroenterology and Digestive Oncology Unit, Avicenne Hospital, HUPSSD, APHP, Université Paris 13, Sorbonne Paris Cité, 125 rue de Stalingrad, Bobigny 93000, France; [b] Gastroenterology and Digestive Oncology Unit, Georges Pompidou Hospital, APHP, Paris Descartes University, 20 Rue Leblanc, Paris 75015, France; [c] Oncology Unit, Saint Antoine Hospital, APHP, 184 Rue du Faubourg Saint-Antoine, Paris 75012, France; [d] Hepato-Gastroenterology Unit, Dijon Hospital, 14 rue Paul Gaffarel, Dijon 21079, France; [e] Translational Cancer Therapeutics department, The Beatson West of Scotland Cancer Centre, University of Glasgow, 1053 Great Western Road, Glasgow G12 0YN, UK
* Corresponding author. Gastroenterology and Digestive Oncology Unit, Avicenne Hospital, APHP, Université Paris 13, Sorbonne Paris Cité, 125 rue de Stalingrad, Bobigny 93000, France.
*E-mail address:* thomas.aparicio@aphp.fr

an adjuvant therapy trial, which is ongoing. Other important information will be obtained from large prospective cohorts.

## EPIDEMIOLOGY
### Small Intestine Cancer

Despite the fact that the small intestine makes up 75% of the length of the digestive tract and 90% of its mucosal surface area, small bowel cancer is rare, accounting for less than 5% of gastrointestinal cancers.[2] According to the National Cancer Data Base (NCDB, 1985-2005) and the Surveillance Epidemiology and End Results (SEER, 1973-2004) database, the incidence of all small bowel cancers in the United States increased from 11.8 cases/million persons in 1973 to 22.7 cases/million persons in 2004.[3] Four histologic types of cancer predominate in the small bowel: adenocarcinomas, neuroendocrine tumors, gastrointestinal stromal tumors and lymphomas.

### Small Bowel Adenocarcinoma

SBA accounts for around 30% to 40% of all cancers of the small intestine.[3–5] The incidence of SBA varies according to geographic location, with higher rates in North America and Western Europe, and lower rates in Asian countries. In the United States, the estimated annual incidence of SBA is about 5300 new cases, with 1100 deaths per year.[6] The median age at diagnosis is in the sixth decade of life, with a sex ratio close to 1. In Europe, the annual incidence is about 5.7 cases per million inhabitants resulting from an estimated number of annual new cases of SBA of 3600 according to the EUROCARE database.[7]

### Duodenum Adenocarcinoma

Duodenum adenocarcinoma is the most common tumor site, as it is seen in more than half of SBA cases, followed by the jejunum and ileum.[3,5,8–11] The increasing incidence of SBA is mainly owing to the increase in duodenum tumors.[12]

## TUMOR PHENOTYPING

Many of the main molecular aberrations that are implicated in the pathogenesis of colorectal cancer have been investigated in SBA (**Table 1**).

### Wnt/Adenomatous polyposis coli /β-Catenin Signaling Pathway
#### Adenomatous polyposis coli

The adenomatous polyposis coli (APC) gene causes a loss of the regulation of β-catenin, which accumulates in the cytoplasm and then in the nucleus and acts as a transcription factor that stimulates the expression of genes involved in cellular proliferation. This mutation is considered one of the main trigger events in colorectal carcinogenesis. The prevalence of the APC gene mutation in SBA is about 10% to 18%[13–16] contrasting to the prevalence of 80% of APC gene mutation observed in colorectal cancer.

#### Nuclear accumulation of β-catenin

Nuclear accumulation of β-catenin, probably caused by a gain-of-function mutation in the β-CATENIN gene, is observed in 20% to 50% of cases.[16–18] Moreover, aberrant activation of the Wnt/β-catenin pathway has been correlated with poor prognosis.[19] Thus, Wnt/β-catenin pathway, even if less common than in colorectal cancer, remains an important pathway for SBA pathogenesis.

**Table 1**
**Molecular abnormalities in small bowel adenocarcinoma**

| Study | N | Abnormal TP53 (%) | Abnormal β−CATENIN (%) | HER2 Overexpression or Mutation (%) | APC Mutation (%) | KRAS Mutation (%) | dMMR Phenotype (%) |
|---|---|---|---|---|---|---|---|
| Laforest et al,[15] 2014 | 83 | 41 | — | 12 | 13 | 43 | 21 |
| Aparicio et al,[17] 2013 | 63 | 42 | 20 | 3.2 | — | 43 | 23 |
| Overman et al,[20] 2010 | 54 | — | — | 1.7 | — | — | 35 |
| Blaker et al,[21] 2004 | 21 | — | 24 | — | 10 | 57 | 7 |
| Svrcek et al,[25] 2003 | 27 | 52 | 7.4 | — | — | — | 18 |
| Planck et al,[27] 2003 | 89 | — | — | — | — | — | 5 |
| Wheeler et al,[16] 2002 | 21 | 24 | 48 | — | 0 | — | 12 |
| Blaker et al,[14] 2002 | 17 | — | — | — | 18 | — | — |
| Nishiyama et al,[22] 2002 | 35 | 40 | — | — | — | 9 | — |
| Arai et al,[13] 1997 | 15 | 27 | — | — | 8 | 53 | — |
| Rashid & Hamilton,[23] 1997 | 22 | — | — | — | — | 40 | 13 |

### Other Tumor Phenotyping

#### Vascular endothelial growth factor and epidermal growth factor receptor

Abnormal expression of vascular endothelial growth factor-A (VEGF-A) and of the epidermal growth factor receptor (EGFR) was found in 50 of 54 (92%) and 36 of 54 (66%) cases, respectively, suggesting that this cancer could benefit from therapies targeting the EGFR and VEGF pathways.[20]

#### RAS

The mutation rate of *KRAS* in SBA is comparable to that observed in colorectal cancers (9%–57%).[13,15,17,21–23] Other *RAS* mutations occur in less than 5% of the tumor.[15]

#### HER2

HER2 protein is rarely overexpressed in contrast to gastric cancer.[17,20] Nevertheless, *HER2* gene mutation or amplification is observed in 12% of SBAs.[15]

#### TP53

*TP53* gene mutation or overexpression of its protein is observed in 24% to 52% of SBAs, suggesting that TP53 plays a major role in this disease.[13,15,16,22,24,25]

### Mismatch Repair Alteration

Inactivation of the DNA mismatch repair (MMR) system is involved in around 15% of colorectal cancers. Deficient MMR (dMMR) can be caused by a germline mutation of one of the 4 MMR genes (usually *MSH2*, or *MLH1*, and more rarely *MSH6* and *PMS2*) as part of Lynch syndrome or to methylation of the *MLH1* promoter in sporadic tumors, especially those occurring in elderly patients in colorectal cancer.[26] In SBA, the frequency of the dMMR phenotype is variable, ranging from 5% to 35% of cases.[14–16,20,23,25,27] Methylation of the MLH1 promoter seems less frequent in dMMR SBA than in dMMR colorectal cancer except in SBA found in association with celiac disease,[28] suggesting that the proportion of Lynch syndrome among dMMR tumors is higher in SBA than in colorectal cancer. The dMMR phenotype was more frequently observed in duodenum and jejunum tumors than in ileum tumors.[15,17]

## RISK FACTORS FOR SMALL BOWEL ADENOCARCINOMA
### Genetic Predisposition

#### Familial adenomatous polyposis

Familial adenomatous polyposis (FAP) is a consequence of a germinal mutation of the *APC* gene. In patient with FAP, SBA is the second most common primary cancer after colorectal cancer. Duodenal adenomas are present in 80% of cases and develop into adenocarcinoma in 4% of cases[29] requiring intensive screening. FAP is present in less than 5% of SBAs.[8] In cases of FAP, SBA occurred mainly in duodenum (71%) or in jejunum (29%).[8]

#### Lynch syndrome

Lynch syndrome is caused by a germline mutation of an MMR gene. In patients with Lynch syndrome, the lifetime cumulative risk for SBA is around 1%.[30] However, an MMR phenotype is systematically recommended in SBA, because it could reveal Lynch syndrome.[31,32] The most common site of SBA in Lynch syndrome is the duodenum (60%), whereas jejunal and ileal locations were reported in 35% and 5% of cases, respectively.[8] The proportion of SBA related to Lynch syndrome is estimated around 6%.[8]

### Peutz-Jeghers syndrome

Peutz-Jeghers syndrome is an autosomal dominant disorder caused by the STK11 suppressor gene mutation that predisposes to hamartomatous gastrointestinal tract polyposis. The estimated cumulative risk of SBA is 13%.[33] The Peutz-Jeghers syndrome is the predisposing disease for less than 1% of SBA.[8]

### Intestinal Diseases

### Crohn's disease

Crohn's disease induces chronic inflammation in the digestive tract. The distal ileum is the site most frequently involved. The chronic inflammation releases cytokines that interact with cell surface receptors and target genes that can promote carcinogenesis.[34] The risk of SBA is correlated with the duration and location of the inflammatory damage. The standardized relative risk compared with the general population is 34 in Crohn's disease affecting the small intestine and 46 for disease duration greater than 8 years.[35] In contrast to SBA in sporadic cases, SBA in Crohn's disease appears in younger patients (fourth decade of life). The cumulative risk is estimated around 0.2% after 10 years and 2.2% after 25 years of Crohn's disease.[36] Crohn's disease is involved in around 8% of SBAs, mostly in ileum.[8]

### Celiac disease

Celiac disease increases the relative risk of SBA from 10 to 30 compared to the general population.[37,38] Celiac disease is associated with SBA in around 2% of cases, the main location is in the jejunum.[8]

### Environmental Factors

In contrast to colorectal cancer, studies of the pathogenesis in SBA are constrained by the rarity of the disease. Alcohol consumption confers a relative risk of around 1.5. Other factors including smoking and consumption of certain foods, such as red meat, sugar, and starchy foods, have been reported to increase the risk of cancer of the small intestine, whereas the consumption of fiber, fruits, vegetables, and fish reduces this risk.[39]

## DIAGNOSIS OF SMALL BOWEL ADENOCARCINOMA

SBA is usually diagnosed in the context of an emergency involving intestinal obstruction or gastrointestinal bleeding. If no source of bleeding has been identified after normal upper and lower endoscopy, several investigations could be considered.

### Computed Tomography with Enteroclysis

Computed tomography with enteroclysis has a sensitivity of between 85% and 95% for the diagnosis of small bowel tumor and a specificity of 90% to 96%.[40,41]

### Video Capsule Endoscopy

Video capsule endoscopy had also a high sensitivity and specificity to detect a small bowel tumor in case of obscure bleeding[42,43] but should not be used in a context of subacute obstruction. A systematic screening for SBA in patients with Lynch syndrome with video capsule endoscopy does not seem to be efficient.[44]

### Double Balloon Enteroscopy

Double balloon enteroscopy can be used to obtain histologic diagnosis.[45]

## PROGNOSIS

SBA carries a poor prognosis. The 5-year overall survival (OS) rate is correlated to the tumor stage: 50% to 60% for stage I, 39% to 55% for stage II, 10% to 40% for stage III, and 3% to 5% for stage IV.[8–11,46,47] SBAs are diagnosed with synchronous metastasis in around 30% of cases, stage III in 30%, stage II in 18% to 27%, and stage I in 5% to 10%.[8,48]

### Lymph Node

Lymph node invasion is the main prognostic factor after resection of localized SBA. In stage III tumor, involvement of ≥3 lymph nodes confers a worse 5-year disease-free survival.[48] For jejuno-ileal tumors, multivariate analysis identified advanced age, advanced stage, an ileal location, the recovery of less than 10 lymph nodes, and the number of positive nodes as significant for poor OS.[49] Thus, a curative resection should systematically include a regional lymphadenectomy.

### Duodenal Primary Tumors

Duodenal primary tumors are associated with worse prognosis in comparison with jejunum and ileum locations.[9,10,48] Other factors have been associated with poor prognosis as advanced age, pT4 tumor stage, poorly differentiated tumor, and positive resection margins.[10,50,51]

### Biologic Factors

Some biological factors are suggested to have prognostic value. A dMMR phenotype is associated with a better disease-fee survival[17] after curative resection. Surprisingly, KRAS mutation is associated with a better survival for patients with metastatic SBA in one study.[17] Mutation of TP53 is associated with poor survival in another study.[24]

### Metastatic Small Bowel Adenocarcinoma

In metastatic SBA treated with chemotherapy, impaired World Health Organization performance status and an above-normal value of carcinoembryonic antigen and carbohydrate antigen 19-9 are prognostic factors for poor survival.[52]

## TREATMENT
### Localized Cancer

#### Surgical resection
Surgical resection (R0) of the primary tumor with loco-regional lymph node resection is the only curative treatment. An R1 or R2 resection should be avoided, as they are associated with a poorer prognosis.[53]

#### Adjuvant chemotherapy
Adjuvant chemotherapy survival benefit has not been found. Several retrospective studies report contradictory results.[1] Despite the lack of evidence supporting the delivery of adjuvant chemotherapy for SBA, an analysis of the National Cancer Database found an increase in the use of chemotherapy from 8% in 1985% to 24% in 2005.[3] However, a prospective international randomized trial (BALLAD study) is ongoing to assess the efficacy of chemotherapy, either fluoropyrimidine monotherapy or combination with oxaliplatin, after R0 resection of stage I–III SBA.

### Metastatic Disease

#### Surgical treatment
Surgical treatment of resectable metastatic SBA is poorly evaluated. A study on 34 patients with resected SBA metastasis reports a median overall survival of 25 months.[54] For unresectable metastatic disease, resection of the primary tumor should be considered in the case of uncontrolled gastrointestinal bleeding, bowel obstruction, or perforation.

#### Palliative chemotherapy
Palliative chemotherapy was evaluated mainly in retrospectives studies[1] (**Table 2**). Median OS ranges from 8 to 22 months and objective response rates (ORR) from 0% to 52%.[52,55–60] Several retrospective studies suggest that chemotherapy offers survival benefit compared with supportive care alone.[9,55,61] Few studies compared chemotherapy regimens. Several retrospectives studies report that gemcitabine- and irinotecan-based chemotherapy are associate with a higher ORR than 5-fluoro-uracil (5FU) monotherapy,[55] platinum-based chemotherapy is associated with a higher ORR and longer median progression-free survival (PFS) than other chemotherapy regimens,[62] the FOLFOX regimen (5FU plus oxaliplatin) is associated with better PFS and OS than 5FU plus cisplatin,[52] and FOLFOX is associated with better PFS and OS than cisplatin- or irinotecan-based regimens.[58] Two prospective phase II studies have evaluated oxaliplatin in combination with 5FU or capecitabine and report an ORR around 50%, a median PFS of 7.8 and 11.3 months, respectively, and median OS of 15.2 and 20.4 months, respectively.[57,63]

**Table 2**
**Studies of chemotherapy for advanced small bowel adenocarcinoma**

| Study | Regimen | N | ORR (%) | PFS (mo) | OS (mo) |
|---|---|---|---|---|---|
| Phase II | | | | | |
| Xiang et al,[63] 2012 | FOLFOX | 33 | 48 | 7.8 | 15.2 |
| Overman et al,[57] 2009 | Capecitabine + oxaliplatine | 30 | 52 | 11.3 | 20.0 |
| Gibson et al,[65] 2005 | 5FU + doxorubicin + MMC | 38 | 18 | 5.0 | 8.0 |
| Retrospective studies | | | | | |
| Tsushima et al,[58] 2012 | 5FU | 60 | 20 | 5.4 | 13.9 |
| | 5FU + cisplatin | 17 | 38 | 3.8 | 12.6 |
| | FOLFOX | 22 | 42 | 8.2 | 22.2 |
| | FOLFIRI | 11 | 25 | 5.6 | 9.4 |
| | Others regimen | 22 | 21 | 3.4 | 8.1 |
| Zaanan et al,[59] 2011 | FOLFIRI (second line) | 28 | 20 | 3.2 | 10.5 |
| Zhang et al,[60] 2011 | Fluoropyrimidine + oxaliplatin | 34 | 32 | 6.3 | 14.2 |
| Zaanan et al,[52] 2010 | FOLFOX | 48 | 34 | 6.9 | 17.8 |
| | 5FU | 10 | 0 | 7.7 | 13.5 |
| | 5FU + cisplatin | 19 | 30 | 6.0 | 9.6 |
| | FOLFIRI | 16 | 9 | 4.8 | 10.6 |
| Overman et al,[62] 2008 | 5FU + cisplatin | 29 | 41 | 8.7 | 14.8 |
| | 5FU without cisplatin | 41 | 17 | 3.9 | 12.0 |
| Fishman et al,[55] 2006 | Various regimens | 44 | 36 | — | — |
| Locher et al,[56] 2005 | 5FU + cisplatin | 20 | 21 | 8.0 | 14.0 |

*Abbreviations:* FOLFIRI, 5FU+irinotecan; MMC, mitomycin C.

### Targeted therapies

Targeted therapies are currently evaluated in phase I or II ongoing studies. A phase II study is currently evaluating first-line chemotherapy with capecitabine plus oxaliplatin in combination with panitumumab (anti-EGFR) in the first-line treatment of SBA without mutation of KRAS (ClinicalTrial.gov identifier: NCT01202409). A phase Ib study is evaluating in the same setting the combination of gemcitabine plus erlotinib (inhibitor of tyrosine kinase of the EGFR) (ClinicalTrial.gov identifier: NCT00987766). A phase II study is evaluating CAPOX chemotherapy plus bevacizumab (NCT01208103). A recent publication shows that inhibition of the anti–programmed death 1 immune checkpoint by pembrolizumab gives dramatic tumor control in patients with dMMR tumors, including 2 SBAs, previously treated with chemotherapy.[64]

## SUMMARY

SBA is a rare cancer. Although certain predisposing factors are now established, most SBAs arise in the absence of risk factors. Studies of molecular abberations suggest that the pathogenesis of SBA is similar to that of colorectal cancer despite fewer *APC* mutations. Surgical resection constitutes the only potentially curative treatment. The margin of resection and nodal invasion are the main prognostic factors. An international prospective, randomized trial is ongoing to assess the benefit of adjuvant chemotherapy (BALLAD study). For patients with advanced SBA, the combination of fluoropyrimidine with oxaliplatin seems to be the most effective systemic chemotherapy regimen, although there are few clinical trials to determine the standard of care. Evaluations of therapies targeting angiogenic or EGFR pathways are ongoing in SBA. Because the incidence of SBA is low, there is a need for development of clinical trials within the framework of international collaborations.

## REFERENCES

1. Aparicio T, Zaanan A, Svrcek M, et al. Small bowel adenocarcinoma: epidemiology, risk factors, diagnosis and treatment. Dig Liver Dis 2013;46:97–104.
2. Neugut AI, Jacobson JS, Suh S, et al. The epidemiology of cancer of the small bowel. Cancer Epidemiol Biomarkers Prev 1998;7:243–51.
3. Bilimoria KY, Bentrem DJ, Wayne JD, et al. Small bowel cancer in the United States: changes in epidemiology, treatment, and survival over the last 20 years. Ann Surg 2009;249:63–71.
4. Jemal A, Siegel R, Ward E, et al. Cancer statistics, 2008. CA Cancer J Clin 2008; 58:71–96.
5. Lepage C, Bouvier AM, Manfredi S, et al. Incidence and management of primary malignant small bowel cancers: a well-defined French population study. Am J Gastroenterol 2006;101:2826–32.
6. Kummar S, Ciesielski TE, Fogarasi MC. Management of small bowel adenocarcinoma. Oncology (Williston Park) 2002;16:1364–9.
7. Faivre J, Trama A, De Angelis R, et al. Incidence, prevalence and survival of patients with rare epithelial digestive cancers diagnosed in Europe in 1995-2002. Eur J Cancer 2012;48:1417–24.
8. Aparicio T, Manfredi S, Tougeron D, et al. A small bowel adenocarcinomas prospective cohort: final analysis of demographic data from nadege study. United European Gastroenterol J 2015;3(S5):A682.
9. Dabaja BS, Suki D, Pro B, et al. Adenocarcinoma of the small bowel: presentation, prognostic factors, and outcome of 217 patients. Cancer 2004;101:518–26.

10. Howe JR, Karnell LH, Menck HR, et al. The American College of Surgeons Commission on Cancer and the American Cancer Society. Adenocarcinoma of the small bowel: review of the National Cancer Data Base, 1985-1995. Cancer 1999;86:2693–706.

11. Moon YW, Rha SY, Shin SJ, et al. Adenocarcinoma of the small bowel at a single Korean institute: management and prognosticators. J Cancer Res Clin Oncol 2010;136:387–94.

12. Chow JS, Chen CC, Ahsan H, et al. A population-based study of the incidence of malignant small bowel tumours: SEER, 1973-1990. Int J Epidemiol 1996;25: 722–8.

13. Arai M, Shimizu S, Imai Y, et al. Mutations of the Ki-ras, p53 and APC genes in adenocarcinomas of the human small intestine. Int J Cancer 1997;70:390–5.

14. Blaker H, von Herbay A, Penzel R, et al. Genetics of adenocarcinomas of the small intestine: frequent deletions at chromosome 18q and mutations of the SMAD4 gene. Oncogene 2002;21:158–64.

15. Laforest A, Aparicio T, Zaanan A, et al. ERBB2 gene as a potential therapeutic target in small bowel adenocarcinoma. Eur J Cancer 2014;50:1740–6.

16. Wheeler JM, Warren BF, Mortensen NJ, et al. An insight into the genetic pathway of adenocarcinoma of the small intestine. Gut 2002;50:218–23.

17. Aparicio T, Svrcek M, Zaanan A, et al. Small bowel adenocarcinoma phenotyping, a clinicobiological prognostic study. Br J Cancer 2013;109:3057–66.

18. Breuhahn K, Singh S, Schirmacher P, et al. Large-scale N-terminal deletions but not point mutations stabilize beta-catenin in small bowel carcinomas, suggesting divergent molecular pathways of small and large intestinal carcinogenesis. J Pathol 2008;215:300–7.

19. Lee HJ, Lee OJ, Jang KT, et al. Combined loss of E-cadherin and aberrant beta-catenin protein expression correlates with a poor prognosis for small intestinal adenocarcinomas. Am J Clin Pathol 2013;139:167–76.

20. Overman MJ, Pozadzides J, Kopetz S, et al. Immunophenotype and molecular characterisation of adenocarcinoma of the small intestine. Br J Cancer 2010; 102:144–50.

21. Blaker H, Helmchen B, Bonisch A, et al. Mutational activation of the RAS-RAF-MAPK and the Wnt pathway in small intestinal adenocarcinomas. Scand J Gastroenterol 2004;39:748–53.

22. Nishiyama K, Yao T, Yonemasu H, et al. Overexpression of p53 protein and point mutation of K-ras genes in primary carcinoma of the small intestine. Oncol Rep 2002;9:293–300.

23. Rashid A, Hamilton SR. Genetic alterations in sporadic and Crohn's-associated adenocarcinomas of the small intestine. Gastroenterology 1997;113:127–35.

24. Alvi MA, McArt DG, Kelly P, et al. Comprehensive molecular pathology analysis of small bowel adenocarcinoma reveals novel targets with potential for clinical utility. Oncotarget 2015;6:20863–74.

25. Svrcek M, Jourdan F, Sebbagh N, et al. Immunohistochemical analysis of adenocarcinoma of the small intestine: a tissue microarray study. J Clin Pathol 2003;56: 898–903.

26. Aparicio T, Schischmanoff O, Poupardin C, et al. Deficient mismatch repair phenotype is a prognostic factor for colorectal cancer in elderly patients. Dig Liver Dis 2012;45(3):245–50.

27. Planck M, Ericson K, Piotrowska Z, et al. Microsatellite instability and expression of MLH1 and MSH2 in carcinomas of the small intestine. Cancer 2003;97:1551–7.

28. Diosdado B, Buffart TE, Watkins R, et al. High-resolution array comparative genomic hybridization in sporadic and celiac disease-related small bowel adeno-carcinomas. Clin Cancer Res 2010;16:1391–401.

29. Vasen HF, Bulow S, Myrhoj T, et al. Decision analysis in the management of duodenal adenomatosis in familial adenomatous polyposis. Gut 1997;40:716–9.

30. Bonadona V, Bonaiti B, Olschwang S, et al. Cancer risks associated with germline mutations in MLH1, MSH2, and MSH6 genes in Lynch syndrome. JAMA 2011; 305:2304–10.

31. Babba T, Schischmanoff O, Lagorce C, et al. Small bowel carcinoma revealing HNPCC syndrome. Gastroenterol Clin Biol 2010;34:325–8.

32. Schulmann K, Brasch FE, Kunstmann E, et al. HNPCC-associated small bowel cancer: clinical and molecular characteristics. Gastroenterology 2005;128:590–9.

33. Giardiello FM, Brensinger JD, Tersmette AC, et al. Very high risk of cancer in fa-milial Peutz-Jeghers syndrome. Gastroenterology 2000;119:1447–53.

34. Schottenfeld D, Beebe-Dimmer JL, Vigneau FD. The epidemiology and patho-genesis of neoplasia in the small intestine. Ann Epidemiol 2009;19:58–69.

35. Elriz K, Carrat F, Carbonnel F, et al. Incidence, presentation, and prognosis of small bowel adenocarcinoma in patients with small bowel Crohn's disease: a pro-spective observational study. Inflamm Bowel Dis 2013;19:1823–6.

36. Palascak-Juif V, Bouvier AM, Cosnes J, et al. Small bowel adenocarcinoma in pa-tients with Crohn's disease compared with small bowel adenocarcinoma de novo. Inflamm Bowel Dis 2005;11:828–32.

37. Askling J, Linet M, Gridley G, et al. Cancer incidence in a population-based cohort of individuals hospitalized with celiac disease or dermatitis herpetiformis. Gastroenterology 2002;123:1428–35.

38. Green PH, Fleischauer AT, Bhagat G, et al. Risk of malignancy in patients with ce-liac disease. Am J Med 2003;115:191–5.

39. Bennett CM, Coleman HG, Veal PG, et al. Lifestyle factors and small intestine adenocarcinoma risk: A systematic review and meta-analysis. Cancer Epidemiol 2015;39:265–73.

40. Boudiaf M, Jaff A, Soyer P, et al. Small-bowel diseases: prospective evaluation of multi-detector row helical CT enteroclysis in 107 consecutive patients. Radiology 2004;233:338–44.

41. Pilleul F, Penigaud M, Milot L, et al. Possible small-bowel neoplasms: contrast-enhanced and water-enhanced multidetector CT enteroclysis. Radiology 2006; 241:796–801.

42. Hartmann D, Schmidt H, Bolz G, et al. A prospective two-center study comparing wireless capsule endoscopy with intraoperative enteroscopy in patients with obscure GI bleeding. Gastrointest Endosc 2005;61:826–32.

43. Pennazio M, Santucci R, Rondonotti E, et al. Outcome of patients with obscure gastrointestinal bleeding after capsule endoscopy: report of 100 consecutive cases. Gastroenterology 2004;126:643–53.

44. Haanstra JF, Al Toma A, Dekker E, et al. Prevalence of small-bowel neoplasia in Lynch syndrome assessed by video capsule endoscopy. Gut 2015;64(10): 1578–83.

45. Hadithi M, Heine GD, Jacobs MA, et al. A prospective study comparing video capsule endoscopy with double-balloon enteroscopy in patients with obscure gastrointestinal bleeding. Am J Gastroenterol 2006;101:52–7.

46. Overman MJ, Hu CY, Kopetz S, et al. A population-based comparison of adeno-carcinoma of the large and small intestine: insights into a rare disease. Ann Surg Oncol 2012;19:1439–45.

47. Talamonti MS, Goetz LH, Rao S, et al. Primary cancers of the small bowel: analysis of prognostic factors and results of surgical management. Arch Surg 2002; 137:564–70.
48. Overman MJ, Hu CY, Wolff RA, et al. Prognostic value of lymph node evaluation in small bowel adenocarcinoma: analysis of the surveillance, epidemiology, and end results database. Cancer 2010;116:5374–82.
49. Nicholl MB, Ahuja V, Conway WC, et al. Small bowel adenocarcinoma: understaged and undertreated? Ann Surg Oncol 2010;17:2728–32.
50. Halfdanarson TR, McWilliams RR, Donohue JH, et al. A single-institution experience with 491 cases of small bowel adenocarcinoma. Am J Surg 2010;199: 797–803.
51. Overman MJ, Kopetz S, Lin E, et al. Is there a role for adjuvant therapy in resected adenocarcinoma of the small intestine. Acta Oncol 2010;49:474–9.
52. Zaanan A, Costes L, Gauthier M, et al. Chemotherapy of advanced small-bowel adenocarcinoma: a multicenter AGEO study. Ann Oncol 2010;21:1786–93.
53. Bakaeen FG, Murr MM, Sarr MG, et al. What prognostic factors are important in duodenal adenocarcinoma? Arch Surg 2000;135:635–41.
54. Rompteaux P, Ganière J, Gornet JM, et al. Métastases d'un adénocarcinome de l'intestin grêle: série de 34 résections. JFHOD 2016.
55. Fishman PN, Pond GR, Moore MJ, et al. Natural history and chemotherapy effectiveness for advanced adenocarcinoma of the small bowel: a retrospective review of 113 cases. Am J Clin Oncol 2006;29:225–31.
56. Locher C, Malka D, Boige V, et al. Combination chemotherapy in advanced small bowel adenocarcinoma. Oncology 2005;69:290–4.
57. Overman MJ, Varadhachary GR, Kopetz S, et al. Phase II study of capecitabine and oxaliplatin for advanced adenocarcinoma of the small bowel and ampulla of vater. J Clin Oncol 2009;27:2598–603.
58. Tsushima T, Taguri M, Honma Y, et al. Multicenter retrospective study of 132 patients with unresectable small bowel adenocarcinoma treated with chemotherapy. Oncologist 2012;17:1163–70.
59. Zaanan A, Gauthier M, Malka D, et al. Second-line chemotherapy with fluorouracil, leucovorin, and irinotecan (FOLFIRI regimen) in patients with advanced small bowel adenocarcinoma after failure of first-line platinum-based chemotherapy: a multicenter AGEO study. Cancer 2011;117:1422–8.
60. Zhang L, Wang LY, Deng YM, et al. Efficacy of the FOLFOX/CAPOX regimen for advanced small bowel adenocarcinoma: a three-center study from China. J BUON 2011;16:689–96.
61. Czaykowski P, Hui D. Chemotherapy in small bowel adenocarcinoma: 10-year experience of the British Columbia Cancer Agency. Clin Oncol (R Coll Radiol) 2007;19:143–9.
62. Overman MJ, Kopetz S, Wen S, et al. Chemotherapy with 5-fluorouracil and a platinum compound improves outcomes in metastatic small bowel adenocarcinoma. Cancer 2008;113:2038–45.
63. Xiang XJ, Liu YW, Zhang L, et al. A phase II study of modified FOLFOX as first-line chemotherapy in advanced small bowel adenocarcinoma. Anticancer Drugs 2012;23:561–6.
64. Le DT, Uram JN, Wang H, et al. PD-1 Blockade in Tumors with Mismatch-Repair Deficiency. N Engl J Med 2015;372:2509–20.
65. Gibson MK, Holcroft CA, Kvols LK, et al. Phase II study of 5-fluorouracil, doxorubicin, and mitomycin C for metastatic small bowel adenocarcinoma. Oncologist 2005;10:132–7.

# Colorectal Cancer
## Genetics is Changing Everything

Joshua C. Obuch, MD[a], Dennis J. Ahnen, MD[b],*

## KEYWORDS

- Colorectal cancer • Genetics • Prevention • Screening • Treatments • Survivorship
- Review

## KEY POINTS

- Impressive declines in incidence and mortality of CRC in the United States have occurred in the last three decades; however, large disparities still exist among African Americans, Hispanics, uninsured, and low-income patients.
- The CIN, MIN, and CIMP pathways are the three main known molecular pathways to colorectal cancer, with each containing different histology, risk factors, prognosis, and response to therapy.
- Further understanding of genetic makeup of CRC has changed the approach to screening and treatment, with targeted therapy options down the pipeline.
- Colonoscopy is the most used CRC screening method in the United States and attention to quality metrics for performance of high-quality colonoscopy is paramount for endoscopists to deliver optimal care.
- Care for patients with CRC extends beyond treatment of the initial tumor. Follow-up care of CRC survivors includes surveillance, counseling regarding posttreatment concerns, and counseling to family members of survivors about their increased cancer risk.

## INTRODUCTION

Cancer is fundamentally a genetic disease caused by mutational or epigenetic alterations in DNA. There has been a remarkable expansion of the molecular understanding of colonic carcinogenesis in the last 30 years and that understanding is changing many aspects of colorectal cancer (CRC) care. This article provides a general update on CRC and highlights how genetics is changing clinical care.

---

Disclosure Statement: J.C. Obuch declares that he has no conflicts of interest. D.J. Ahnen has received board membership payments and paid travel accommodations from EXACT Sciences, Inc, board membership payments from Cancer Prevention Pharmaceuticals, and a speaker's honorarium from Ambry Genetics. Scientific Advisory Board EXACT Sciences; Scientific Advisory Board Cancer Prevention Pharmaceuticals; Speakers Bureau Ambry Genetics.

[a] Division of Gastroenterology & Hepatology, Department of Medicine, University of Colorado, School of Medicine, 12631 E. 17th Avenue, MS B-158, Aurora, CO 80045, USA; [b] University of Colorado, School of Medicine, 12631 E. 17th Avenue, MS B-158, Aurora, CO 80045, USA
* Corresponding author.
*E-mail address:* dennis.ahnen@ucdenver.edu

Gastroenterol Clin N Am 45 (2016) 459–476
http://dx.doi.org/10.1016/j.gtc.2016.04.005
0889-8553/16/$ – see front matter © 2016 Elsevier Inc. All rights reserved.

## MOLECULAR PATHWAYS

The molecular understanding of colonic carcinogenesis continues to rapidly evolve (**Fig. 1**). Both hereditary and sporadic CRCs are genetically driven diseases. Hereditary CRC syndromes are caused by germline mutations and sporadic CRC is driven by alterations in DNA structure (mutations) or function (epigenetics).

# Molecular Pathways to Colorectal Cancer

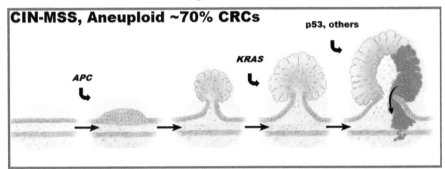

**CIN-MSS, Aneuploid ~70% CRCs**

p53, others

KRAS

APC

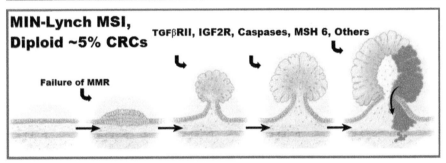

**MIN-Lynch MSI, Diploid ~5% CRCs**

TGFβRII, IGF2R, Caspases, MSH 6, Others

Failure of MMR

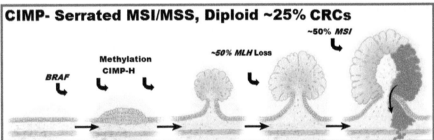

**CIMP- Serrated MSI/MSS, Diploid ~25% CRCs**

~50% MSI

~50% MLH Loss

Methylation
CIMP-H

BRAF

**Fig. 1.** Molecular pathways to CRC. The chromosomal instability (CIN) pathway (*top*) is driven by sequential mutational events (activating mutations in oncogenes, such as *KRAS*, and inactivating mutations in tumor suppressor genes, such as *APC* or *p53*) and leads to CRCs that are typically aneuploid, microsatellite stable (MSS), and may have KRAS but not BRAF mutations. The microsatellite instability (MIN) pathway (*middle*) is caused by germline mutations in one of the DNA mismatch repair genes and leads to Lynch syndrome CRCs, which are hypermutated, have microsatellite instability (MSI), and may have KRAS but not BRAF mutations. The CpG island methylator phenotype (CIMP) or serrated pathway leads to CRCs that are MSI or MSS and often have BRAF but not KRAS mutations. These molecular pathways have different histology, prognosis, and response to therapy. (*Adapted from* Janne PA, Mayer RJ. Chemoprevention of colorectal cancer. N Engl J Med 2000;342(26):1961.)

About 6% of all CRCs are caused by a hereditary syndrome for which the genetic basis has been identified. Germline mutations in more than 15 genes that are required for DNA repair and/or regulation of signaling pathways that affect DNA repair are now known to cause an increased risk of CRC. These syndromes can be nonpolyposis syndromes, such as Lynch syndrome, or can be colonic polyposis syndromes with development of scores to thousands of adenomatous, hamartomatous, and/or serrated polyps (**Table 1**).

The three major pathways to CRC (chromosomal instability [CIN], microsatellite instability (MIN)/Lynch, and CpG island methylator phenotype [CIMP]/serrated) are described in **Fig. 1**. Both the CIN and MIN pathways are thought to progress through the classic adenoma-carcinoma sequence, whereas the CIMP pathway is a serrated polyp-carcinoma sequence. As a first approximation, CRCs from these pathways are distinguished based on microsatellite stability (MSS) and the mutational status of KRAS and BRAF as shown in **Fig. 1** but this is an oversimplification: the mutational/epigenetic composition of CRCs is highly varied with the average CRC containing around 90 different mutations.[1] The Cancer Genome Atlas separated CRCs into hypermutated (16% of CRCs; median mutation number, 728) and nonhypermutated (median of 58 mutations) groups and found that the mutational profiles of the groups differ.[2] Several more complex classification systems are being developed in hopes of more precisely predicting biologic behavior and response to therapy.[3] It is becoming increasingly clear that there are genetic subsets of CRCs that have different risk factors, prognosis, and response to treatment. This article highlights how the genetic understanding of CRC is changing almost all facets of CRC care.

## PUBLIC HEALTH BURDEN

The global incidence of CRC was estimated to be about 1.4 million in 2012; it is the third most common cancer worldwide accounting for about 10% of the total cancer burden.[4] There is up to a 10-fold difference in CRC incidence and mortality around

**Table 1**
**Hereditary colorectal cancer syndromes**

| Syndrome | Genes | Functions |
|---|---|---|
| Lynch syndrome | MLH-1, MSH-2, MSH-6, PMS-2 EPCAM | Required for DNA mismatch repair |
| Familial adenomatous polyposis | APC | Regulates Wnt signaling |
| MUTYH-associated polyposis | MUTYH | Required for DNA base excision repair |
| Proofreading polymerase-associated polyposis | POLD1, POLE | Required for proofreading and repair of polymerase errors during DNA replication |
| Hereditary mixed polyposis | GREM1 | Bone morphogenic protein antagonist, regulates transforming growth factor-β signaling |
| Familial juvenile polyposis | SMAD4, BMPR1 | Regulates transforming growth factor-β signaling |
| Peutz-Jeghers syndrome | STK-11 | Kinase that regulates multiple signaling pathways |
| Cowden disease, Bannayan-Riley-Ruvalcaba syndrome | PTEN | Negative regulator of AKT signaling |
| CHEK2 | CHEK2 | Negative regulator of cyclin-dependent kinases |

the world,[5] with higher rates generally found in high-income countries. Time trends show incidence and mortality are continuing to increase in low-income countries but have stabilized or are declining in many high-income countries.

There has been an impressive decline in the United States over the last 30 years in the incidence (36%) and mortality (50%) of CRC (**Fig. 2**) that has been attributed largely to CRC screening. Nonetheless, CRC remains the fourth most common cancer (>134,000 cases) and second leading cause of cancer-related mortality (>49,000 deaths) in the United States[6,7] with substantial demographic disparities in CRC outcomes.

CRC rates are decreasing in all age groups except those younger than age 50 where an increase in rectal cancer has been seen.[8] Reports from Surveillance, Epidemiology, and End Results CRC registry data initially identified concerning increased incidence of young adult CRCs with an annual percentage increase of about 1.5% to 2% for patients 20 to 49 years of age.[9,10]

African Americans have the poorest CRC outcomes in the United States,[11] are diagnosed at a later stage of disease,[12] and have about a 10% lower 5-year survival than white persons.[13] These disparities are thought to be largely caused by differences in access to care. In 2012, 70% of white persons compared with 66% of African Americans aged 50 and older ever had a screening colonoscopy or sigmoidoscopy. Similarly, screening rates are lower among Hispanics (56.8%) and persons with annual incomes less than $15,000 (53.8%).[14] For uninsured individuals, screening rates are

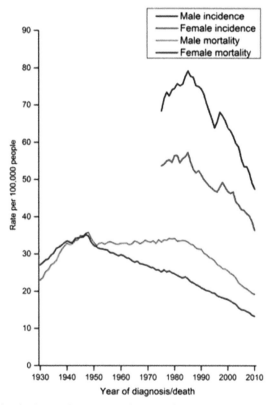

**Fig. 2.** Time trends of colorectal cancer incidence and mortality in the United States. (*From* Siegel R, Desantis C, Jemal A. Colorectal cancer statistics, 2014. CA Cancer J Clin 2014;64(2):112; with permission.)

particularly low, with one study citing 33% of uninsured patients undergoing any test for CRC screening compared with 77% of insured patients.[15] The identification of geographic "hotspots" of high CRC mortality within the United States by Siegel and colleagues[16] may be caused by poverty and racially driven decreased access to care.

### Impact of Genetics on Colorectal Cancer Burden

Genetic factors play an important role in CRC risk and predisposition. Not only is CRC driven by genetic and epigenetic alterations in DNA (see **Fig. 1**), about 25% of patients with CRC have a family history of the disease (familial CRC) and about 6% of CRCs are caused by a defined hereditary syndrome. Currently germline mutations in more than 15 different genes (see **Table 1**) have been shown to cause hereditary CRC. It is now recognized that there is substantial clinical overlap between CRC hereditary syndromes, such as Lynch syndrome, and hereditary breast and ovarian cancer syndrome[17] and that the phenotype of several polyposis syndromes overlap substantially. This, along with the dramatically decreasing costs of next-generation sequencing, has led to a marked increase in cancer gene panel use to assess high-risk families, which in turn has improved the understanding of the phenotypic expression of these genetic syndromes. Genome-wide association studies have identified at least 23 single-nucleotide polymorphisms that are associated with modest increases in CRC risk.[18] Lastly, it is likely that gene-environment interactions are responsible for at least some of the risk in the remaining families with multiple CRCs.

## RISK AND PROTECTIVE FACTORS

Increasing age, male sex, African American race, and birth/residence in high-income countries are well established nonmodifiable risk factors for CRC. Although observational studies have consistently reported obesity, lack of physical activity, alcohol/tobacco use, and diets high in red/processed meats and low in fruits/vegetables/fiber are associated with an increased CRC risk,[19] it is not clear to what extent changing these risk factors in an adult modulates risk. Nonetheless, prevention recommendations for CRC (**Box 1**) are similar to those for cardiovascular disease prevention and seem prudent.

### Impact of Genetics

Genetic factors not only influence the likelihood of developing many of these risk factors (obesity, alcohol and tobacco use),[20–22] but undoubtedly also modulate the risk of

---

**Box 1**
**Recommendations for CRC prevention**

Get screened

Avoid tobacco

Limit alcohol consumption

Stay lean

Get regular physical activity

Limit red meat intake

Avoid processed meat

Increase intake of fiber-containing foods including fruits and vegetables

Consider aspirin if you are also at high risk for cardiovascular disease

CRC development in individuals with these risk factors. Among a large number of potential chemopreventive approaches,[23] the strongest body of evidence supports aspirin use and other nonsteroidal anti-inflammatory drugs in this setting.[24–30] A large number of observational and interventional studies have shown long-term aspirin use is associated with substantial (20%–40%) decreases in sporadic adenoma incidence,[31] metachronous adenoma incidence,[32] sporadic CRC incidence, and mortality[33,34] and a decreased risk of metastases in CRCs.[35] The beneficial effects of aspirin on colonic carcinogenesis seem to be modulated by genetic susceptibility. Nan and colleagues[36] showed the protective effect of aspirin differed dramatically as a function of two single-nucleotide polymorphisms at chromosomes 12 and 15. Observational studies have also suggested that aspirin may improve overall survival in patients with CRC, with the effect being more pronounced in PIK3CA mutated tumors. Liao and colleagues[28] reported a dramatic survival effect of aspirin use in patients with PIK3CA mutant with an HR for CRC-specific survival of 0.18 (0.06–0.61) and overall survival of 0.54 (95% confidence interval, 0.31–0.94), with no effect in patients with PIK3CA wild-type CRCs (hazard ratio, 0.96; 95% confidence interval, 0.69–1.32; and hazard ratio, 0.94; 95% confidence interval, 0.75–1.17, respectively). A recent systematic review and meta-analysis found heterogeneity in the results but concluded the benefit of postdiagnosis aspirin treatment on overall mortality in CRC is more pronounced in PIK3CA mutated tumors.[29]

## SCREENING AND EARLY DETECTION

CRC screening is the standard of care in the United States. The US Preventive Services Task Force[37] and all the gastrointestinal and cancer societies recommend colon cancer screening in the general population starting by age 50 (some recommend by age 45 in African Americans) (**Table 2**). Screening for CRC can prevent CRC by identification and removal of colonic polyps in addition to early detection of CRCs. The concept of precancerous polyps eventually giving rise to CRC was suggested as early as 1927.[38] The recognition by Dukes in 1932[39] that CRC survival was better in earlier stage disease birthed the notion that removal of precancerous polyps and detection of early stage CRC could reduce the impact of CRC. The history of CRC screening has been recently chronicled,[40] and indeed much of the recent decline in CRC incidence and mortality in the United States (see **Fig. 2**) is thought to be caused by these efforts.

CRC screening is discussed in detail elsewhere in this issue (see Anderson BW, Ahlquist, DA: Molecular Detection of Gastrointestinal Neoplasia: Innovations in Early Detection and Screening, in this issue) but the current status of screening tests is summarized here. CRC screening tests recommended in the United States are divided into those that primarily detect cancer (fecal occult blood tests [FOBT], fecal immunochemical tests [FIT], stool DNA tests) and those that can also detect polyps (flexible sigmoidoscopy [FS], colonoscopy, computed tomography colonography). Multiple controlled trials have shown that guaiac-based FOBTs decrease CRC mortality by 12% to 33%.[41] Although FITs have not been studied in controlled trials with cancer mortality as the end point, they are preferred over guaiac-based FOBTs based on their higher sensitivity for CRC.[41] Stool DNA tests, in turn, have a higher sensitivity but lower specificity than FITs for CRC and advanced adenomas.[42]

FS has been shown in controlled trials to reduce CRC mortality by about 25%.[41] Despite a lack of controlled trials, case-control and cohort studies have indicated superiority of colonoscopy over FS, making colonoscopy the preferred intervention because of its higher sensitivity for CRC and adenoma detection compared with FS. Several controlled trials are currently underway comparing the effectiveness of

**Table 2**
**Colorectal cancer screening tests**

| Colon Cancer Prevention Screening | 2008 USMSTF Followup Recommendations | 2015 USPSTF Followup Recommendations |
|---|---|---|
| Flexible Sigmoidoscopy | 5 y (+/− FOBT or FIT every y) | 5 y or every 10 y + Annual FIT |
| Colonoscopy | 10 y | 10 y |
| Double Contrast Balloon Enema | 5 y | Not recommended |
| CT Colonography | 5 y | 5 y |
| **Colon Cancer Detection Screening** | | |
| High Sensitivity Guiac Fecal Occult Blood Test or High Sensitivity Fecal Immunochemistry Test | Annual | Annual |
| Stool DNA Test | Interval Uncertain | 1 or 3 y[a] |

*Abbreviations:* FIT, fecal immunochemical tests; FOBT, fecal occult blood tests; USMSTF, US Multisociety Task Force; USPSTF, US Preventive Services Task Force.

[a] Interval recommended by manufacturer.

*From* United States Preventative Services Task Force. Draft Recommendation Statement: Colorectal Cancer: Screening. 2015. Available at: http://www.uspreventiveservicestaskforce.org/Page/Document/draft-recommendation-statement38/colorectal-cancer-screening2. Accessed December 20, 2015.

colonoscopy to FOBTs including one in the United States (the CONFIRM trial in the United States funded by the Veterans Administration [ClinicalTrials.gov NCT01239082]); the final results of these trials are still a decade away.

Although arguments can be made for which CRC screening test is superior, the best screening test is the one that gets done and done well. Determinants of which screening options are feasible in a country depends largely on health resource availability. The World Gastroenterology Organization has outlined a resource-based cascade of CRC screening options to provide a framework for health care systems to do the best with the available resources and the Organization is actively engaged in many countries to promote affordable screening options and provide training in endoscopic skills in low-resource countries.[43]

Although there are quality issues relevant to all CRC screening tests, colonoscopy is thought to be the most operator-dependent. Thus, substantial efforts have been made to improve colonoscopy quality.[44] Missed adenomas are thought to be the most common reason for interval CRCs (CRCs that occur before the next recommended screening examination). The adenoma detection rate (ADR), which is the fraction of patients undergoing screening colonoscopy who had one or more adenomas detected, inversely correlates with interval CRC risk[45,46] and has been adopted by the American College of Gastroenterology and American Society for Gastrointestinal Endoscopy as perhaps the most important quality indicator in screening colonoscopy. The initial targets for ADR (25% for men; 15% for women) were set at levels slightly below the mean detection rates of adenomas in screening colonoscopy studies.[47,48] ADRs have been increasing progressively with improvements in colonoscopic equipment, preparation quality, and endoscopic technique; recent studies report many endoscopists have ADRs exceeding 40%[49,50] or even 50%.[51,52] Based on these data, recommended ADR targets were recently revised to 30% for men and 20% for women.[53]

Endoscopists with ADRs less than 25% should take steps to improve their ADR. One predictor of a low ADR is short withdrawal time (WT; time of mucosal inspection during withdrawal of the scope from the cecum).[54,55] It is recommended that WTs be recorded as a colonoscopy quality measure and that average WT should be 6 minutes or more in screening colonoscopies. Endoscopists with low ADRs and short WTs should slow down and take more time to inspect the colonic mucosa and improve their technique (examining proximal portion of folds, suctioning pools of liquid, adequate distention of the colonic lumen). Although incomplete resection of polyps is also thought to be an important contributor to interval cancers,[56] quality measures have not yet address this issue.

### Impact of Genetics on Colorectal Cancer Screening

Genetic factors have long been used to stratify risk, modify screening recommendations, and recently genetic screening for sporadic CRCs has become available. Screening recommendations for genetically defined hereditary CRC syndromes typically involve much more intense screening regimens often with annual colonoscopy starting in adolescence or young adulthood.[57] Similarly, individuals with one first-degree relative with CRC younger than age 60 or greater than one first-degree relative with CRC but no identifiable hereditary syndrome are advised to use colonoscopy every 5 years as the preferred screening strategy and to start screening at age 40 or 5 to 10 years younger than the earliest CRC in the family. A recent study[58] reported that patients with a family history of CRC had modestly higher overall screening rates than those without, but screening rates in the 40 to 49 age group in high-risk families was less than 40%, leaving substantial room for improvement.

The first DNA-based test was recently approved by the Food and Drug Administration and Centers for Medicare/Medicaid Services for CRC screening in the general population based on a large controlled trial[59] showing that a multitarget stool test that includes FIT and a panel of genetic and methylated DNA markers (Cologuard) was superior to FIT alone for detecting CRCs (sensitivity, 92% vs 74%) and advanced adenomas (sensitivity, 42% vs 24%). A blood test for methylated septin 9 is clinically available for CRC screening in Europe and parts of Asia with a reported 85% sensitivity for CRC but a low sensitivity for advanced adenomas ($\approx$20%).[60] Additional blood-based genetic screening tests are currently in development.

Screening protocols and effectiveness of CRC screening vary as a function of the molecular basis of the CRC. The adenoma-carcinoma sequence progresses more rapidly in the microsatellite instability (MSI)/Lynch pathway so colonoscopy screening is recommended more frequently (1–2 years regardless if polyps are found).[57] CRC screening also seems to be less effective for MSI CRCs (arising from either the MIN/Lynch or the CIMP/serrated pathway; see **Fig. 1**); MSI is two to three times more common in interval CRCs than in noninterval CRCs,[61] although it is not clear whether this is caused by more rapid progression of this pathway or that serrated polyps are more difficult to identify and remove compared with conventional adenomas.[62]

## DIAGNOSTIC EVALUATION

CRC is usually diagnosed by evaluation of symptoms or conventional screening. Rectal bleeding, change in bowel habits, and abdominal pain are the most common symptoms in patients with CRC (>40% sensitivity) with bleeding and altered bowel habits more common in proximal cancers and identifiable rectal bleeding more common in distal cancers. These symptoms are also common in other gastrointestinal conditions and their positive predictive value for CRC is low (<10%).[63] Both patients and providers often attribute these symptoms to other conditions leading to diagnostic delay. This is a particularly common issue in young adults in whom CRC is less common. CRCs in young adults are often advanced when detected, with one study[64] citing more than 58% of patients presenting with stage III or IV disease. Thus inclusion of CRC in the differential diagnosis of these symptoms, particularly when they are persistent or progressive, is important.[65]

CRC is increasingly being diagnosed by screening, and colonoscopy is central to this diagnosis either as the initial screening examination or follow-up examination to another positive screening test. The diagnostic accuracy of colonoscopy is critically dependent on the quality of the colonoscopic examination. However, there is substantial variability in the quality of colonoscopy among endoscopists[44] primarily because of differences in endoscopic technique, training, and experience. The American Society for Gastrointestinal Endoscopy and American College of Gastroenterology have adopted quality thresholds for colonoscopy[53] including ADR, WT, bowel preparation, and cecal intubation rates (**Table 3**).

Bowel preparation is particularly important to the effectiveness of colonoscopic diagnosis of CRC; it can be quantitatively measured using the Boston Bowel Preparation Scale[66] or Ottawa Bowel Preparation scale[67]; ultimately colonoscopic evaluation is considered adequate if it allows detection of polyps greater than 5 mm in size.[47] Vigorous bowel cleansing during colonoscopy may be needed to allow adequate mucosal inspection; if bowel cleansing is still inadequate the procedure is considered suboptimal and should be repeated.[68] Split dose bowel preparation with half the preparation the night before and the remainder the morning of the procedure improves preparation quality and patient tolerance.[69] For afternoon colonoscopies, a morning preparation completed at least 2 hours before sedation is an effective option.[70]

Complete colonoscopy requires cecal intubation (ie, passage of the colonoscope proximal to the ileocecal valve); incomplete colonoscopy has been associated with increased rates of interval proximal CRC.[71] High-quality endoscopists should have overall cecal intubation rates greater than 90% and greater than 95% for CRC screenings or surveillance examinations; photo documentation of cecal landmarks should confirm a complete examination.[42,72,73] Given the higher incidence of interval CRCs in the proximal colon and greater difficulty in detecting right sided polyps, many experts recommend a "second look" at the right colon with or without cecal retroflexion.[74,75]

| Table 3 Quality metrics in endoscopy | |
|---|---|
| **Metric** | **Goal** |
| Frequency of adequate bowel preparation to allow use of recommended surveillance or screening intervals | ≥85% of outpatient examinations |
| Cecal intubation rate | ≥90% of all examinations |
| Adenoma detection rate in average risk screening examinations | ≥25% (men ≥30%, women ≥20%) |
| Average withdrawal time on a negative screening colonoscopy | ≥6 min |

*Data from* Rex DK, Schoenfield PS, Cohen J, et al. Quality indicators for colonoscopy. Am J Gastroenterol 2015;110(1):72–90.

## Impact of Genetics on Colorectal Cancer Diagnosis

CRCs that arise through the MSI/Lynch and CIMP/serrated pathways may be more difficult to diagnose than those that arise through the CIN pathway because, like their precursor polyps, they are more common in the proximal colon, can be endoscopically more subtle, and may progress from polyps to cancer quickly.[56]

## PROGNOSIS

Classically the prognosis of CRC has been defined by the pathologic stage of the disease defined by the TNM staging system.[76] Five-year survival ranges from about 75% to 90% for stage I disease (tumor confined to bowel wall, no lymph node or metastatic disease) to 6% for stage IV (metastatic) disease. Histologic features, such as grade, degree of differentiation, and lymphovascular invasion may influence prognosis but are not routinely included in the TNM staging system.

## Impact of Genetics

Molecular features have been shown to be powerful prognostic markers for CRC.[77] MSI CRCs, regardless if they arise through the MSI/Lynch or CIMP/serrated pathway, have a better prognosis than MSS tumors.[78] Conversely BRAF mutation in MSS CRCs is a marker of worse prognosis.[79] Phipps and colleagues[80] reported that even after adjusting for disease stage MSI CRCs arising from the MSI/Lynch or CIMP/serrated pathway had substantially better 5-year survival (>80%) than MSS/KRAS mutant (68%) cancers and BRAF mutant CRCs had the worst survival (46%).

## CLINICAL MANAGEMENT

High-quality surgical resection is the basis of all potentially curative therapy for CRC. The type of resection depends on several factors including location, size, stage of CRC, patient preference, and surgical expertise. It is generally recognized that laparoscopic resection in expert hands is oncologically equivalent to open resection for colon cancer, and total mesorectal excision should be the routine approach for rectal cancer resection,[81] with better outcomes when performed by high-volume surgeons at high-volume centers.[82,83]

Chemotherapeutic approaches have expanded greatly in the last decade.[84] 5-Fluorouracil (5-FU; with or without leucovorin or levamisol) has been used for CRC chemotherapy since the 1960s and was essentially the only option for 40 years. Since 2004, a total of 10 new drugs have received Food and Drug Administration approval for treatment of CRC (**Table 4**).

For stage II colon cancer, adjuvant therapy is controversial; its use is individualized based on clinical comorbidities, details of TNM staging, and histologic (poorly differentiated, neural invasion) and genetic (MSI status) features. Stage III colon cancers routinely use adjuvant chemotherapy, which has been shown to reduce recurrence and mortality by 20% to 30%, and combinations of 5-FU or capecitabine plus oxaliplatin with or without leucovorin is generally recommended as first-line therapy.

For stage II or early stage III rectal cancer, postoperative therapy with a combination of chemotherapy (typically a fluoropyrimidine and oxalaplatin) and radiation with fluoropyrimidine radiosenstization is done. Neoadjuvant chemoradiotherapy is typically recommended for stage III rectal cancers with evidence of transmural involvement on rectal endoscopic ultrasound or MRI.

First-line chemotherapy for metastatic CRC includes combinations of a fluoropyrimidine (5-FU, capecitabine, or trifluorident-tiparacil) with either oxalaplatin or

**Table 4**
**FDA-approved chemotherapeutic agents in the United States**

|  | Class | Mechanism | FDA Approved |
|---|---|---|---|
| 5-FU[a] | Cytotoxic antimetabolite | Inhibition of thymidylate synthetase | 1962 |
| Bevacizumab | Monoclonal antibody | Blocks VEGF | 2004 |
| Cetuximab | Monoclonal antibody | Blocks EGF receptor signaling | 2004 |
| Panitumumab | Monoclonal antibody | Blocks EGF receptor signaling | 2006 |
| Irinotecan | Cytotoxic | Topoisomerase inhibitor leads to double-stranded DNA breaks | 2008 |
| Oxaliplatin | Cytotoxic Alkylating agent | Binds to DNA, induces DNA cross-links | 2009 |
| Regorofanib | Oral angiogenesis inhibitor | Blocks multiple kinases including VEGF signaling | 2012 |
| Afibercept | Fusion protein Angiogenesis inhibitor | Decoy receptor, blocks binding to multiple receptors including VEGF | 2012 |
| Capecitabine | Oral cytotoxic antimetabolite | Oral 5-FU, inhibition of thymidylate synthetase | 2013 |
| Ramucirumab | Monoclonal antibody | Blocks VEGF receptor | 2015 |
| Trifluridint-tipiracil | Oral cytotoxic antimetabolite | Inhibition of thymidylate synthetase and thymidine phosphorylase | 2015 |

*Abbreviations:* EGF, epidermal growth factor; FDA, Food and Drug Administration; VEGF, vascular endothelial growth factor.
[a] Usually given with *leucovorin* [LV].
*Data from* Gustavsson B, Carlsson G, Machover D, et al. A review of the evolution of systemic chemotherapy in the management of colorectal cancer. Clin Colorectal Cancer 2015;14(1):1–10.

irinotecan. The addition of the angiogenesis inhibitor bevacizumab or anti–epidermal growth factor receptor antibodies (cetuximab, pentulimamab) is also used as first-line therapy for selected populations.

### Impact of Genetics

Specific genetic features of CRC predict survival and response to therapy. MSI CRCs have the best and MSS/BRAF mutant CRCs have the worst survival.[80] Patients with stage II MSI colon cancers have a very good prognosis and should not be treated with adjuvant therapy. MSI CRCs do not respond to adjuvant therapy with 5-FU alone, although they do respond to 5-FU plus oxalaplatin. The findings that KRAS and BRAF mutant CRCs do not respond to anti–epidermal growth factor receptor therapy[85] has allowed targeting of these expensive agents to patients who are more likely to benefit.

MSI CRCs are hypermutated[2]; it is thought their improved prognosis is caused by an enhanced Th1 cytotoxic immunologic response to expression of numerous mutation-related neoantigens. The programmed death 1 pathway, a negative feedback system that represses prolonged Th1 cytotoxic immune responses, could blunt the immunologic response to CRCs. A recent uncontrolled trial in heavily pretreated patients with metastatic disease reported MSI, but not MSS, CRCs showed marked radiologic and serologic response to the anti–programmed death 1 inhibitor pembrolizumab.[86] If confirmed, this observation will launch a new era in molecularly targeted therapy for CRCs.

Many laboratories are using molecular markers of CRCs to identify potential therapeutic targets in patients who have failed conventional therapy. Whether this approach improves outcomes is not clear.

## SURVIVORSHIP

There are more than 1 million CRC survivors in the United States.[87] Multifaceted care including surveillance for recurrence and new cancers, management and monitoring of treatment effects, and promotion of healthy lifestyle behaviors is required for survivors (**Table 5**).[88] Although substantial progress has been made in the medical management of CRC survivors, survivor concerns and health information needs, such as tests/treatments, health promotion, side effects, symptoms, and interpersonal/emotional issues of survivors recently completing treatment, have not been addressed as aggressively.[89] In a qualitative study by Sterba and colleagues,[89] survivors received complex surveillance care with multiple providers and frequent tests. However, they did not receive assistance in actively transitioning from treatment to the posttreatment period, suggesting a need for development of formal educational survivorship interventions focused on provision of tools and resources at the end of treatment to facilitate a better understanding of expectations and positive transitions at the end of treatment.

**Table 5**
**CRC surveillance guidelines**

|  | 1–2 y Postresection | 2–5 y Postresection |
|---|---|---|
| **Rectal cancer surveillance guidelines** |  |  |
| History and physical | 3–6 mo | 6 mo |
| CEA | 3–6 mo | 6 mo |
| CT chest/abdomen/pelvis | 3–6 mo | 6–12 mo |
| Proctoscopy (with EUS or MRI)[a] | 3–6 mo | 6 mo |
| Colonoscopy | 1 y postresection (3–6 mo if no preoperative colonoscopy because of obstruction) If advanced adenoma, repeat in 1 y If no advanced adenomas, repeat in 3 y then every 5 y |  |
| **Colon cancer surveillance guidelines** |  |  |
| History and physical | 3–6 mo | 6 mo |
| CEA | 3–6 mo | 6 mo |
| CT chest/abdomen/pelvis | 6–12 mo | 6–12 mo |
| Colonoscopy | 1 y postresection (3–6 mo if no preoperative colonoscopy because of obstruction) If advanced adenoma, repeat in 1 y If no advanced adenomas, repeat in 3 y then every 5 y |  |

*Abbreviations:* CEA, carcinoembryonic antigen; CT, computed tomography; EUS, endoscopic ultrasound.
   [a] Patient with transanal excision only.
   *Data from* National Comprehensive Cancer Network. National Comprehensive Cancer Network practice guidelines in oncology: colon cancer version 3.2015. 2015. Available at: http://www.nccn.org/professionals/physician_gls/f_guidelines.asp#site. Accessed October 13, 2015.

Tan and colleagues[90] surveyed a group of CRC survivors annually over the course of their survivorship and reported that, particularly in women, concerns regarding recurrence of their cancer were highest 1 year after cure, with concerns shifting toward ways of reducing the risk of family members from developing the same or different cancer in the ensuing years. Indeed, family members of CRC survivors are at increased risk of developing CRC and other cancers.[91] As part of a "survivor package", patients should be provided with not only instructions on what to expect and how to better manage their life, but also information to provide to their close relatives about their CRC risk.

### Impact of Genetics

CRC survivors are key to identification of familial and hereditary CRC. Close relatives of CRC survivors are at increased risk of the disease and the risk increases directly with the number of close relatives with CRC and inversely with both the age of the CRC in the survivor and that of the relative.[92] Similarly, universal testing of CRCs for MSI will identify Lynch syndrome in some survivors, information that is critically important for their family members. Survivors have a unique opportunity to help their family by ensuring family members are aware of their cancer, informing the family about other members that have had cancers and the results of any genetic testing that was performed/recommended, and ensuring that their family members talk to their own medical providers about CRC screening at least 10 years before the earliest CRC in the family. In this way, survivors play a critical role to prevent CRC in their families.

The ongoing revolution in the molecular understanding of colonic carcinogenesis has had a major impact on almost every aspect of CRC care. Hereditary syndromes contribute significantly to the public health burden of CRC. Molecular factors modulate susceptibility to CRC risk factors and benefit from chemoprevention and even effectiveness of CRC screening. Similarly, CRC prognosis and treatment responses are dependent on the molecular profile of CRCs. Finally, CRC survivors are key to the identification of high-risk families. It is likely that even the classification of CRC will evolve to include molecular designations (ie, MSI CRC). Vive la révolution!

## REFERENCES

1. Sjoblom T, Jones S, Wood LD, et al. The consensus coding sequences of human breast and colorectal cancers. Science 2006;314(5797):268–74.
2. Cancer Genome Atlas Network. Comprehensive molecular characterization of human colon and rectal cancer. Nature 2012;487(7407):330–7.
3. Biswas S, Holyoake D, Maughan TS. Molecular taxonomy and tumourigenesis of colorectal cancer. Clin Oncol (R Coll Radiol) 2016;28(2):73–82.
4. World Health Organization. GLOBOCAN 2012: estimated cancer incidence, mortality, and prevalence worldwide in 2012. 2012. Available at: http://globocan.iarc.fr/Pages/summary_table_pop_sel.aspx. Accessed September 8, 2015.
5. Arnold M, Sierra MS, Laversanne M, et al. Global patterns and trends in colorectal cancer incidence and mortality. Gut 2016;0:1–9.
6. National Cancer Institute. A snapshot of colorectal cancer. 2014. Available at: http://www.cancer.gov/research/progress/snapshots/colorectal. Accessed September 8, 2015.
7. Siegel RL, Miller KD, Jemal A. Cancer statistics, 2016. CA Cancer J Clin 2016;66(1):7–30.
8. Scott RB, Rangel LE, Osler TM, et al. Rectal cancer in patients under the age of 50 years: the delayed diagnosis. Am J Surg 2015;211(6):1014–8.

9. Siegel RL, Jemal A, Ward EM. Increase in incidence of colorectal cancer among young men and women in the United States. Cancer Epidemiol Biomarkers Prev 2009;18(6):1695–8.

10. O'Connell JB, Maggard MA, Liu JH, et al. Rates of colon and rectal cancers are increasing in young adults. Am Surg 2003;69(10):866–72.

11. Siegel RL, Desantis C, Jemal A. Colorectal cancer statistics, 2014. CA Cancer J Clin 2014;64(2):104–17.

12. Shipp MP, Desmond R, Accortt N, et al. Population-based study of the geographic variation in colon cancer incidence in Alabama: relationship to socio-economic status indicators and physician density. South Med J 2005;98(11): 1076–82.

13. Silber JH, Rosenbaum PR, Ross RN, et al. Racial disparities in colon cancer survival: a matched cohort study. Ann Intern Med 2014;161(12):845–54.

14. Center for Disease Control. Behavioral risk factor surveillance system. 2013. Available at: http://www.cdc.gov/brfss. Accessed December 20, 2015.

15. Matthews BA, Anderson RC, Nattinger AB. Colorectal cancer screening behavior and health insurance status (United States). Cancer Causes Control 2005;16(6): 735–42.

16. Siegel RL, Sahar L, Robbins A, et al. Where can colorectal cancer screening interventions have the most impact? Cancer Epidemiol Biomarkers Prev 2015; 24(8):1151–6.

17. Yurgelun MB, Allen B, Kaldate RR, et al. Identification of a variety of mutations in cancer predisposition genes in patients with suspected lynch syndrome. Gastroenterology 2015;149(3):604–13.

18. Whiffin N, Hosking FJ, Farrington SM, et al. Identification of susceptibility loci for colorectal cancer in a genome-wide meta-analysis. Hum Mol Genet 2014;23(17): 4729–37.

19. Bouvard V, Loomis D, Guyton KZ, et al. Carcinogenicity of consumption of red and processed meat. Lancet Oncol 2015;16(16):1599–600.

20. Dick DM, Agrawal A. The genetics of alcohol and other drug dependence. Alcohol Res Health 2008;31(2):111–8.

21. Treutlein J, Strohmaier J, Frank J, et al. Smoking behaviour: investigation of the coaction of environmental and genetic risk factors. Psychiatr Genet 2014;24(6): 279–80.

22. Walley AJ, Blakemore AI, Froguel P. Genetics of obesity and the prediction of risk for health. Hum Mol Genet 2006;15(Spec No 2):R124–30.

23. Crosara Teixeira M, Braghiroli MI, Sabbaga J, et al. Primary prevention of colorectal cancer: myth or reality? World J Gastroenterol 2014;20(41):15060–9.

24. Chubak J, Kamineni A, Buist DSM, et al. U.S. preventive services task force evidence syntheses, formerly systematic evidence reviews, in aspirin use for the prevention of colorectal cancer: an updated systematic evidence review for the U.S. Preventive Services Task Force. Rockville (MD): Agency for Healthcare Research and Quality (US); 2015.

25. Domingo E, Church DN, Sieber O, et al. Evaluation of PIK3CA mutation as a predictor of benefit from nonsteroidal anti-inflammatory drug therapy in colorectal cancer. J Clin Oncol 2013;31(34):4297–305.

26. Fajardo AM, Piazza GA. Chemoprevention in gastrointestinal physiology and disease. Anti-inflammatory approaches for colorectal cancer chemoprevention. Am J Physiol Gastrointest Liver Physiol 2015;309(2):G59–70.

27. Kothari N, Kim R, Jorissen RN, et al. Impact of regular aspirin use on overall and cancer-specific survival in patients with colorectal cancer harboring a PIK3CA mutation. Acta Oncol 2015;54(4):487–92.

28. Liao X, Lochhead P, Nishihara R, et al. Aspirin use, tumor PIK3CA mutation, and colorectal-cancer survival. N Engl J Med 2012;367(17):1596–606.

29. Paleari L, Puntoni M, Clavarezza M, et al. PIK3CA mutation, aspirin use after diagnosis and survival of colorectal cancer. A systematic review and meta-analysis of epidemiological studies. Clin Oncol (R Coll Radiol) 2016;28(5):317–26.

30. Chae YK, Kim K, Hong D, et al. PIK3CA mutation, aspirin use and mortality in patients with metastatic colorectal cancer participating in early-phase clinical trials. Abstract. Proceedings of the 104th Annual Meeting of the American Association for Cancer Research Cancer Res, Cancer Res 2013;73:164.

31. Hawk ET, Limburg PJ, Viner JL. Epidemiology and prevention of colorectal cancer. Surg Clin North Am 2002;82(5):905–41.

32. Wang Y, Zhang FC, Wang YJ. The efficacy and safety of non-steroidal anti-inflammatory drugs in preventing the recurrence of colorectal adenoma: a meta-analysis and systematic review of randomized trials. Colorectal Dis 2015;17(3): 188–96.

33. Rothwell PM, Wilson M, Elwin CE, et al. Long-term effect of aspirin on colorectal cancer incidence and mortality: 20-year follow-up of five randomised trials. Lancet 2010;376(9754):1741–50.

34. Rothwell PM, Fowkes FG, Belch JF, et al. Effect of daily aspirin on long-term risk of death due to cancer: analysis of individual patient data from randomised trials. Lancet 2011;377(9759):31–41.

35. Rothwell PM, Wilson M, Price JF, et al. Effect of daily aspirin on risk of cancer metastasis: a study of incident cancers during randomised controlled trials. Lancet 2012;379(9826):1591–601.

36. Nan H, Hutter CM, Lin Y, et al. Association of aspirin and NSAID use with risk of colorectal cancer according to genetic variants. JAMA 2015;313(11):1133–42.

37. United States Preventative Services Task Force. Draft recommendation statement: colorectal cancer: screening. 2015. Available at: http://www.uspreventiveservicestaskforce.org/Page/Document/UpdateSummaryFinal/colorectal-cancer-screening2?ds=1&s=colon%20cancer. Accessed March 16, 2016.

38. Lockhart-Mummery JP, Dukes C. The precancerous changes in the rectum and colon. Surg Gynecol Obstet 1927;36:591–6.

39. Dukes C. The classification of cancer of the rectum. J Pathol Bacteriol 1932;35: 323–32.

40. Winawer SJ. The history of colorectal cancer screening: a personal perspective. Dig Dis Sci 2015;60(3):596–608.

41. Leung WC, Foo DC, Chan TT, et al. Alternatives to colonoscopy for population-wide colorectal cancer screening. Hong Kong Med J 2016;22(1):70–7.

42. Imperiale TF, Wagner DR, Lin CY, et al. Risk of advanced proximal neoplasms in asymptomatic adults according to the distal colorectal findings. N Engl J Med 2000;343(3):169–74.

43. Winawer SJ, Krabshuis J, Lambert R, et al, World Gastroenterology Organization Guidelines Committee. Cascade colorectal cancer screening guidelines: a global conceptual model. J Clin Gastroenterol 2011;45(4):297–300.

44. Fayad NF, Kahi CJ. Colonoscopy quality assessment. Gastrointest Endosc Clin N Am 2015;25(2):373–86.

45. Kaminski MF, Regula J, Kraszewska E, et al. Quality indicators for colonoscopy and the risk of interval cancer. N Engl J Med 2010;362(19):1795–803.

46. Corley DA, Jensen CD, Marks AR, et al. Adenoma detection rate and risk of colorectal cancer and death. N Engl J Med 2014;370(14):1298–306.

47. Rex DK, Bond JH, Winawer S, et al. Quality in the technical performance of colonoscopy and the continuous quality improvement process for colonoscopy: recommendations of the U.S. Multi-Society Task Force on Colorectal Cancer. Am J Gastroenterol 2002;97(6):1296–308.

48. Rex DK, Petrini JL, Baron TH, et al. Quality indicators for colonoscopy. Am J Gastroenterol 2006;101(4):873–85.

49. Barclay RL, Vicari JJ, Doughty AS, et al. Colonoscopic withdrawal times and adenoma detection during screening colonoscopy. N Engl J Med 2006;355(24):2533–41.

50. Chen SC, Rex DK. Endoscopist can be more powerful than age and male gender in predicting adenoma detection at colonoscopy. Am J Gastroenterol 2007;102(4):856–61.

51. Kahi CJ, Anderson JC, Waxman I, et al. High-definition chromocolonoscopy vs. high-definition white light colonoscopy for average-risk colorectal cancer screening. Am J Gastroenterol 2010;105(6):1301–7.

52. Rex DK, Helbig CC. High yields of small and flat adenomas with high-definition colonoscopes using either white light or narrow band imaging. Gastroenterology 2007;133(1):42–7.

53. Rex DK, Schoenfield PS, Cohen J, et al. Quality indicators for colonoscopy. Am J Gastroenterol 2015;110(1):72–90.

54. Lee RH, Tang RS, Muthusamy VR, et al. Quality of colonoscopy withdrawal technique and variability in adenoma detection rates (with videos). Gastrointest Endosc 2011;74(1):128–34.

55. Rex DK. Colonoscopic withdrawal technique is associated with adenoma miss rates. Gastrointest Endosc 2000;51(1):33–6.

56. Patel SG, Ahnen DJ. Prevention of interval colorectal cancers: what every clinician needs to know. Clin Gastroenterol Hepatol 2014;12(1):7–15.

57. Syngal S, Brand RE, Church JM, et al. ACG clinical guideline: genetic testing and management of hereditary gastrointestinal cancer syndromes. Am J Gastroenterol 2015;110(2):223–62.

58. Tsai MH, Xirasagar S, Li YJ, et al. Colonoscopy screening among US adults aged 40 or older with a family history of colorectal cancer. Prev Chronic Dis 2015;12:E80.

59. Imperiale TF, Ransohoff DF, Itzkowitz SH, et al. Multitarget stool DNA testing for colorectal-cancer screening. N Engl J Med 2014;370(14):1287–97.

60. Epigenomics. 2016. Available at: http://www.epigenomics.com/en/products-services/epi-procolon.html. Accessed January 10, 2016.

61. Cisyk AL, Singh H, McManus KJ. Establishing a biological profile for interval colorectal cancers. Dig Dis Sci 2014;59(10):2390–402.

62. Obuch JC, Pigott CM, Ahnen DJ. Sessile serrated polyps: detection, eradication, and prevention of the evil twin. Curr Treat Options Gastroenterol 2015;13(1):156–70.

63. Vega P, Valentin F, Cubiella J. Colorectal cancer diagnosis: pitfalls and opportunities. World J Gastrointest Oncol 2015;7(12):422–33.

64. Liang J, Kalady MF, Church J. Young age of onset colorectal cancers. Int J Colorectal Dis 2015;30(12):1653–7.

65. Ahnen DJ, Wade SW, Jones WF, et al. The increasing incidence of young-onset colorectal cancer: a call to action. Mayo Clin Proc 2014;89(2):216–24.

66. Calderwood AH, Jacobson BC. Comprehensive validation of the Boston bowel preparation scale. Gastrointest Endosc 2010;72(4):686–92.

67. Rostom A, Jolicoeur E. Validation of a new scale for the assessment of bowel preparation quality. Gastrointest Endosc 2004;59(4):482–6.

68. Lieberman DA, Rex DK, Winawer SJ, et al. Guidelines for colonoscopy surveillance after screening and polypectomy: a consensus update by the US Multi-Society Task Force on Colorectal Cancer. Gastroenterology 2012;143(3):844–57.

69. Kilgore TW, Abdinoor AA, Szary NM, et al. Bowel preparation with split-dose polyethylene glycol before colonoscopy: a meta-analysis of randomized controlled trials. Gastrointest Endosc 2011;73(6):1240–5.

70. Varughese S, Kumar AR, George A, et al. Morning-only one-gallon polyethylene glycol improves bowel cleansing for afternoon colonoscopies: a randomized endoscopist-blinded prospective study. Am J Gastroenterol 2010;105(11):2368–74.

71. Baxter NN, Sutradhar R, Forbes SS, et al. Analysis of administrative data finds endoscopist quality measures associated with postcolonoscopy colorectal cancer. Gastroenterology 2011;140(1):65–72.

72. Kadakia SC, Wrobleski CS, Kadakia AS, et al. Prevalence of proximal colonic polyps in average-risk asymptomatic patients with negative fecal occult blood tests and flexible sigmoidoscopy. Gastrointest Endosc 1996;44(2):112–7.

73. Rathgaber SW, Wick TM. Colonoscopy completion and complication rates in a community gastroenterology practice. Gastrointest Endosc 2006;64(4):556–62.

74. Harrison M, Singh N, Rex DK. Impact of proximal colon retroflexion on adenoma miss rates. Am J Gastroenterol 2004;99(3):519–22.

75. Hewett DG, Rex DK. Miss rate of right-sided colon examination during colonoscopy defined by retroflexion: an observational study. Gastrointest Endosc 2011;74(2):246–52.

76. Edge S, Byrd DR, Compton CC, et al. AJCC cancer staging manual. 7th edition. New York: Springer-Verlag New York; 2010. p. 648.

77. Sideris M, Papagrigoriadis S. Molecular biomarkers and classification models in the evaluation of the prognosis of colorectal cancer. Anticancer Res 2014;34(5):2061–8.

78. Popat S, Hubner R, Houlston RS. Systematic review of microsatellite instability and colorectal cancer prognosis. J Clin Oncol 2005;23(3):609–18.

79. Clarke CN, Kopetz ES. BRAF mutant colorectal cancer as a distinct subset of colorectal cancer: clinical characteristics, clinical behavior, and response to targeted therapies. J Gastrointest Oncol 2015;6(6):660–7.

80. Phipps AI, Limburg PJ, Baron JA, et al. Association between molecular subtypes of colorectal cancer and patient survival. Gastroenterology 2015;148(1):77–87.

81. Tjandra JJ, Kilkenny JW, Buie WD, et al. Practice parameters for the management of rectal cancer (revised). Dis Colon Rectum 2005;48(3):411–23.

82. Archampong D, Borowski D, Wille-Jorgensen P, et al. Workload and surgeon's specialty for outcome after colorectal cancer surgery. Cochrane Database Syst Rev 2012;(3):CD005391.

83. Merlino J. Defining the volume-quality debate: is it the surgeon, the center, or the training? Clin Colon Rectal Surg 2007;20(3):231–6.

84. Gustavsson B, Carlsson G, Machover D, et al. A review of the evolution of systemic chemotherapy in the management of colorectal cancer. Clin Colorectal Cancer 2015;14(1):1–10.

85. Kirstein MM, Lange A, Prenzler A, et al. Targeted therapies in metastatic colorectal cancer: a systematic review and assessment of currently available data. Oncologist 2014;19(11):1156–68.

86. Le DT, Uram JN, Wang H, et al. PD-1 blockade in tumors with mismatch-repair deficiency. N Engl J Med 2015;372(26):2509–20.

87. American Cancer Society. Cancer facts & figures 2014. 2014. Available at: http://www.cancer.org/cancer/colonandrectumcancer/detailedguide/colorectal-cancer-key-statistics. Accessed October 11, 2015.

88. National Comprehensive Cancer Network. National comprehensive cancer network practice guidelines in oncology: colon cancer version 3.2015. 2015. Available at: http://www.nccn.org/professionals/physician_gls/f_guidelines.asp#site. Accessed October 13, 2015.

89. Sterba KR, Zapka J, LaPelle N, et al. A formative study of colon cancer surveillance care: implications for survivor-centered interventions. J Cancer Educ 2015;30(4):719–27.

90. Tan AS, Nagler RH, Hornik RC, et al. Evolving information needs among colon, breast, and prostate cancer survivors: results from a longitudinal mixed-effects analysis. Cancer Epidemiol Biomarkers Prev 2015;24(7):1071–8.

91. Samadder NJ, Jasperson K, Burt RW. Hereditary and common familial colorectal cancer: evidence for colorectal screening. Dig Dis Sci 2015;60(3):734–47.

92. Samadder NJ, Smith KR, Hanson H, et al. Increased risk of colorectal cancer among family members of all ages, regardless of age of index case at diagnosis. Clin Gastroenterol Hepatol 2015;13(13):2305–11.

# Knowns and Known Unknowns of Gastrointestinal Stromal Tumor Adjuvant Therapy

Virginia Martínez-Marín, MD, PhD[a], Robert G. Maki, MD, PhD[b],*

## KEYWORDS

- Gastrointestinal stromal tumor (GIST) • *KIT* mutation • *PDGFRA* mutation
- Adjuvant therapy • Imatinib

## KEY POINTS

- For higher-risk primary gastrointestinal stromal tumor (GIST), 3 years of imatinib in the adjuvant setting is the standard of care.
- Neoadjuvant therapy with imatinib can shrink very large primary tumors to make surgery easier later, but such GIST should be considered very high-risk tumors.
- Specific genetic subtypes such as such as those GIST without *KIT* or *PDGFRA* mutation do not benefit from adjuvant imatinib therapy, based on inherent resistance to imatinib of some genomic GIST subtype; others do not merit adjuvant therapy due to their lower risk of recurrence.
- Reimaging in follow-up should take into account the risk of recurrence on and after the completion of adjuvant treatment.

## INTRODUCTION

The first 15 years of active therapy of gastrointestinal stromal tumor (GIST) set the stage for the development of treatment of solid tumors, thanks to small molecule oral kinase inhibitors such as imatinib. The discovery of *KIT* mutations in GIST[1] led to the understanding of KIT as a driver of GIST growth and has led to the understanding of the clonal evolution of a solid tumor over time.[2] Imatinib as a KIT inhibitor in GIST

Conflicts of Interest: None (V. Martínez-Marín); Consulting or clinical trials support: American Board of Internal Medicine, Sarcoma Alliance for Research through Collaboration (SARC), Arcus, Bayer, Eisai/Morphotek, Gem Pharmaceuticals, GSK, Lilly/Imclone, Novartis, Pfizer (R.G. Maki).
[a] Medical Oncology Service, Hospital Universitario La Paz, P° de la Castellana, 261, Madrid 28046, Spain; [b] Tisch Cancer Institute, Department of Medicine, Mt Sinai Medical Center, 1 Gus Levy Place, New York, NY 10029-6574, USA
* Corresponding author.
*E-mail address:* robert.maki@mssm.edu

Gastroenterol Clin N Am 45 (2016) 477–486
http://dx.doi.org/10.1016/j.gtc.2016.04.006
0889-8553/16/$ – see front matter © 2016 Elsevier Inc. All rights reserved.

in vitro[3] and in people with metastatic disease[4,5] sparked a wave of activity leading to approval of 3 agents in many countries for metastatic GIST, specifically imatinib, sunitinib, and regorafenib.[6–8] In parallel with the developments in metastatic disease, a series of clinical trials has been conducted that led to the present standard of care after resection of higher-risk GIST, specifically 3 years of imatinib.[9]

Despite an apparently complete and coherent set of data outlining therapy for primary and metastatic disease, patients still progress despite all lines of therapy, indicating the need for further research on adapting treatment as metastatic disease evolves. In addition, several issues remain regarding the use of 3 years of imatinib in the adjuvant setting. It is this latter series of questions that is addressed in this review.

Adjuvant imatinib therapy has been observed applied blindly to patients with larger tumors with higher mitotic rates. However, the genetics of GISTs, which has impact on the treatment of metastatic disease, also contributes to the decision making of who should receive adjuvant therapy. These data are still evolving and remain one of the most interesting issues of the "first-order" problems in GIST management. The treatment of large primary tumors in which neoadjuvant imatinib is used preoperatively is also an important area of clinical interest, in which there is some practical experience. Finally, how many scans are necessary to help most efficiently identify recurrence in patients who have either not received or have received adjuvant therapy? The kinetics of recurrence has important implications for patient care as well.

It is hoped that in this review that some of these evolving "knowns" and "known unknowns" in the adjuvant therapy of GIST are addressed, so that clinicians can contribute to the next series of studies that will better define the role of adjuvant therapy for GIST.

## CASE SERIES FROM THE ERA BEFORE IMATINIB THERAPY

It was clear from older series of GIST patients that there was a significant recurrence and death rate from recurrent disease. In the oldest large series from MD Anderson, Ng and colleagues[10] showed that what was then called gastrointestinal leiomyosarcoma had a very high recurrence and mortality risk. A series of 200 GIST patients from Memorial Sloan Kettering Cancer Center showed a high recurrence and disease-specific death rate.[11] Notably, both of these series involved patients with larger tumors than is seen in more contemporary series of primary disease. GIST proved unyielding to standard cytotoxic chemotherapy, for reasons that remain unknown.[12] As a result, the finding of patients with metastatic disease responding to imatinib quickly led to the implementation of adjuvant trials to attempt to improve the cure rate.

Joensuu and colleagues[13] have compiled the largest retrospective analysis of GIST involving patients from the era before imatinib, which in addition to data from Z9000[14] and Z9001[15] discussed later, form the basis of discussion of the risk of recurrence of GIST on the specific mutation driving the tumor. The Z9000 and Z9001 genetic data also allow at least some insight into the impact of imatinib on these relatively small subsets of patients.

From a population of more than 3000 GIST patients, mutation analysis was conducted in 1505 of the patients. Relapse-free survival (RFS) was the principal endpoint for the analysis. A total of 301 unique *KIT* mutations and 33 *PDGFRA* mutations were observed. The most common mutations overall were deletion of WK557-558 (*KIT* exon 11), substitution of D842V (*PDGFRA* exon 18), and duplication of AY502-503 (*KIT* exon 9). These mutations were associated with a similar RFS to other GISTs.[13]

Although mitotic rate still was more important than genomic status of the GIST in terms of prognosis, specific genetic subtypes were associated with better outcomes than others. In particular, patients with *PDGFRA* mutations had superior RFS compared with GISTs with *KIT* mutations (hazard ratio [HR], 0.34; $P = .004$).

Looking specifically at *KIT*-mutated GIST, patients with *KIT* exon 9 mutated GIST showed a numerically inferior PFS compared with *KIT* exon 11 mutated GIST ($P = .07$).[13] Approximately 80% of *KIT* exon 9 mutations were seen in small bowel GIST. In terms of rarer *KIT* mutant GISTs, both primary exon 13 and 17 primary GISTs were nongastric and did not portend a different prognosis than other *KIT* mutant GIST.[13]

Notably, some subtypes of *KIT* exon 11 mutations were substantially lower-risk tumors than the most common mutation subtypes. For example, only 1 in 35 GISTs with *KIT* exon 11 duplication mutations recurred. Patients with deletions of only one codon of *KIT* exon 11 had better RFS than those with another deletion type, and specific *KIT* exon 11 substitution mutations (W557R, V559A, and L576P) were also associated with better RFS. Patients with no *KIT* or *PDGFRA* mutation also had a lower risk of recurrence compared with all patients (HR 0.52; $P<.001$). Eighty-eight percent of *PDGFRA* mutations were found in gastric GISTs.

These data form the foundation of the expected genomic subtypes by location, which recur at different rates after surgery, impacting who recurs after therapy, be it surgery, imatinib, or both.

## SELECTED TRIALS OF ADJUVANT IMATINIB

The key trial of imatinib in the adjuvant setting that has led to the 2016 standard of care of 3-year imatinib for higher-risk GIST is discussed after setting the stage discussing other important trials.

### Z9000 (1-YEAR IMATINIB)

Two trials led by DeMatteo with the American College of Surgeons Oncology Group, trials Z9000 (phase II)[14] and Z9001 (phase III),[15] led to the approval of imatinib in the adjuvant setting.

The Z9000 study of imatinib 400 mg oral daily for 1 year after resection of primary high-risk GIST was heartening, whereby high risk was defined as tumor diameter of 10 cm or more, intraperitoneal tumor rupture, or up to 4 peritoneal implants. A total of 106 people were treated. With a median follow-up of 7.7 years, RFS rates were 96%, 60%, and 40% at 1, 3, and 5 years, respectively. Overall survival (OS) rates were 99%, 97%, and 83%, much better than historical 5-year OS rates of 35%.[14]

The *KIT* and *PDGFRA* mutation data from Z9000 confirmed the higher-risk nature of *KIT* exon 11 deletion mutations compared with other mutation classes. *KIT* exon 11 mutant GIST patients had clear benefit from imatinib overall.[14] Patients with *KIT* exon 9 mutant GIST had approximately the same relapse risk with or without imatinib, calling into question the use of imatinib in this group of GIST. Conversely, in the European Organisation for Research and Treatment of Cancer metastatic disease study discussed later, higher doses of imatinib appear to be more effective in the metastatic setting, suggesting higher-dose therapy for *KIT* exon 9 mutant GIST if it is to be used. Patients without *KIT* or *PDGFRA* mutations appear to have no difference in RFS regardless of whether they received imatinib or not, implying that such patients are not good candidates for adjuvant imatinib. Finally, patients with *PDGFRA* mutation other than D842V appeared to benefit; the very low risk of recurrence of and the resistance of such GIST to imatinib are 2 reasons to not use adjuvant imatinib in *PDGFRA* D842V patients (see later discussion).

## Z9001 (0 VS 1-YEAR ADJUVANT IMATINIB)

The Z9001 was the first trial to compare imatinib and placebo in the adjuvant setting, testing 1 year of treatment.[15,16] A total of 713 patients with resected primary localized GIST at least 3 cm in greatest dimension were treated. In the initial analysis with median follow-up of ∼20 months, RFS was superior with imatinib versus placebo (98% vs 83%; $P<.001$). OS was not different (99.2% vs 99.7%; $P = .47$). The benefit of imatinib could be stratified by tumor size, with RFS in favor of treatment only for larger tumors (for 6–10 cm size tumors, RFS was 98% for imatinib vs 76% for placebo; $P = .05$); the difference in RFS was greater for primary GISTs >10 cm in size (77% versus 41%; $P<.0001$).

The most recent follow-up of the Z9001 focused on genetic data and their impact on outcomes in the trial.[15] With a median follow-up of 74 months, RFS remained superior for 1 year of imatinib (HR 0.6; 95% CI 0.43–0.75). Examining the control and imatinib arms separately, in each case by multivariate analysis, the tumor genotype was not significantly associated with RFS in comparison with the known significant factors of larger tumor, small bowel location, and high mitotic rate. OS was not impacted by 1 year of imatinib; patients with relapse did well for extended periods of time on imatinib after relapse.

Comparing the 2 arms of the trial, imatinib was associated with superior RFS in patients with *KIT* exon 11 deletion, but not *KIT* exon 11 insertion or point mutation, *KIT* exon 9 mutations, *PDGFRA* mutation, or for tumors without *PDGFRA* or *KIT* mutation.

## EUROPEAN ORGANISATION FOR RESEARCH AND TREATMENT OF CANCER INTERGROUP TRIAL (0 VS 2-YEAR ADJUVANT IMATINIB)

A large international study examined 2 versus 0 years of imatinib in the adjuvant setting for intermediate- to high-risk resected GIST, using the novel endpoint of failure of first tyrosine kinase inhibitor as a primary endpoint, meaning that patients had to fail imatinib in the adjuvant and recurrent setting to be declared a failure.[17] Eight hundred thirty-five eligible patients were accrued internationally. With 4.7-year median follow-up, 5-year imatinib failure-free survival was not different (97% for imatinib vs 84% for placebo), and OS was essentially identical (100% for imatinib vs 99% for placebo), but RFS was significantly different at 3 years (84% vs 66%) and at 5 years (69% vs 63%) ($P<.001$). The data across these studies are consistent with the relapse of patients most commonly 6 to 18 months after completion of adjuvant therapy. These data were supported by a smaller phase II trial of 2 years of imatinib for *KIT* exon 11 mutant GIST from Korea, with consistent data.[18]

## SCANDINAVIAN SARCOMA GROUP XVIII/ARBEITSGEMEINSCHAFT INTERNISTISCHE ONKOLOGIE (1 VS 3-YEAR ADJUVANT IMATINIB)

The study that defines present day adjuvant therapy for GIST is the Scandinavian Sarcoma Group (SSG) XVIII/Arbeitsgemeinschaft Internistische Onkologie (AIO) trial of 3 years of imatinib versus 1 year of imatinib, in which both RFS and OS were superior for 3 years of imatinib versus 1 year.[9] Two hundred evaluable patients were treated on each arm, and all had higher-risk disease as defined by having at least 1 of the following features: (1) longest tumor diameter greater than 10 cm, (2) mitotic rate greater than 10 per 50 high-power fields (HPF) of the microscope, (3) tumor diameter greater than 5.0 cm and mitotic count greater than 5/50 HPF, or (4) tumor rupture before surgery or at surgery. With a median follow-up of 54 months, RFS was superior for 3-year imatinib, 66% versus 48% ($P<.0001$); 5-year OS was 92% versus 82% in favor of 3-year imatinib ($P$ = .019). In a 2016 follow-up analysis with median follow up of 90 months, 5-year RFS was 71% for imatinib versus 52% for placebo, and 5-year OS was 92% versus 85%.[19] Mutation analysis of this group of patients, not published as of the 2016 update, will provide a unique resource as to who should or should not receive adjuvant imatinib on the basis of their mutation status and other known risk factors.

## ONGOING ADJUVANT TRIALS

There are 2 important ongoing adjuvant trials to examine the question of longer duration of therapy. One is the phase II trial PERSIST-5 of 5 years of imatinib to assess the upper bounds of benefit of longer duration imatinib; this study completed accrual and the study data are maturing (see Clinicaltrials.gov identifier NCT00867113). SSG XXII is a follow-up study to SSG XVIII. SSG XXII is a randomized trial of 3-year versus 5-year study through the SSG and collaborating organizations. The latter study is limited to the highest-risk tumors, defined as gastric GIST with mitotic count greater than 10/50 HPF, or nongastric GIST with mitotic count greater than 5/50 HPF, or tumor presenting with rupture (NCT02413736).

## NEOADJUVANT THERAPY

There is a single phase II study of neoadjuvant and adjuvant imatinib, which involved both patients with primary and metastatic GIST. In this study, RTOG 0132, preoperative imatinib was given initially at 600 mg orally daily for approximately 2 months and then continued postoperatively for 2 years.[20,21] At the most recent published analysis, median follow-up was 5.1 years. Focusing on the 31 patients with primary disease only, estimated 5-year RFS was 57%, and OS was 77%.[20] Genetic data for this study have not been published to date.

It is fairly clear that for patients with high-risk GIST, in particular very large tumors greater than 15 cm with high mitotic rates, recurrence rates are very high after stopping neoadjuvant imatinib. It may well be that microscopic disease remains in the tumor bed after tumor shrinking. The authors thus generally maintain imatinib postoperatively to complete at least 3 years of therapy and typically consider such patients to have at least microscopic metastatic disease from the time of diagnosis. There are data from some difficult primary sites (eg, rectum) that local control rate may be better with imatinib in the neoadjuvant setting than without it.[22]

## REIMAGING

For more common cancers, it is not clear that any specific schedule of screening for recurrence helps to improve survival. Responsible clinicians want to expose their patients to as few procedures as possible. In this light, how many scans are enough to detect GIST recurrences? Joensuu and colleagues,[23] modeling the SSG XVIII/AIO data, provided insight in the form of the risk of relapse as a function of time after starting and stopping the 3 years of adjuvant therapy. National Comprehensive Cancer Network (NCCN) guidelines, discussed further later, suggest computed tomographic (CT) imaging every 3 to 6 months for 3 to 5 years and then annually.[24] In the SSG XVIII trial, relatively few people relapse on adjuvant therapy; however, the period of time 6 to 18 months after stopping imatinib appears to the highest risk time for GIST recurrence. These data lead to at least one modified recommendation, for CT or MRI every 6 months during adjuvant imatinib, every 3 to 4 months during the 2 years after discontinuation of imatinib, and then at 6- to 12-month intervals to complete 10 years of follow-up.[25] Recurrence after the first 10 years of follow-up is infrequent. Modified recommendations for reimaging of patients with GIST with lower risk who do not receive imatinib are also available.

## SENSITIVITY OF GASTROINTESTINAL STROMAL TUMOR–SPECIFIC *KIT* AND *PDGFRA* MUTATIONS TO IMATINIB

It has been clear for more than a decade that different mutations in GIST will predict for better or worse outcomes in metastatic disease. These clinical data are buttressed by data from GIST cell lines or transfection experiments of cell lines bearing different forms of mutated *KIT* or *PDGFRA* molecules. An attempt to condense 15 years of data on gene mutation and imatinib sensitivity in the metastatic setting in vivo and in vitro is presented in **Table 1**. In short, the in vitro testing of imatinib in GIST cell lines or *KIT* or *PDGFRA* mutant transfectants does not appear to be a good means to determine sensitivity to imatinib clinically, but do appear to correlate more strongly with imatinib resistance when observed in vitro.

By virtue of the data in **Table 1**, given the lack of sensitivity of *PDGFRA* D842V GIST in vitro and in the metastatic setting clinically, imatinib is not indicated in the adjuvant setting for such patients. In a similar fashion, GIST that do not have *KIT* or *PDGFRA* mutation do not appear to be good candidates for adjuvant imatinib. It is also difficult to suggest imatinib for rare variants that appear to be resistant to imatinib in the metastatic setting or in vitro.

## NATIONAL AND INTERNATIONAL GUIDELINES

The European Society for Medical Oncology (ESMO) and NCCN guidelines both present similar recommendations for adjuvant therapy,[24,26] with the ESMO guidelines perhaps more granular. The ESMO guidelines follow the criteria of the SSG XVIII study for the selection of patients appropriate for adjuvant imatinib, exclude *PDGFRA* D842V and *NF1* mutant GIST patients, and note controversy over succinate dehydrogenase (SDH) deficient GIST. The authors support the notion of no adjuvant therapy for SDH-mutant GIST given their indolent phenotype in most patients and lack of response seen with metastatic disease to imatinib. These data argue that the reason people do well with SDH-deficient GIST is not from the result of drug but rather the natural history of the diagnosis.

## COMMENTARY

The data regarding mutations and sensitivity or resistance to imatinib colors the choice of patients to treat with adjuvant therapy for GIST. Patients with *PDGFRA* D842V, *NF1*, *BRAF*, and (the authors would argue) SDH loss do not have partial responses to imatinib in the metastatic setting and thus appear to be inappropriate candidates for imatinib. The scenario of imatinib resistance may also play out clinically for other GIST mutation classes, for example, *KIT* L576P or exon 12 mutations. The molecular data from the SSG XVIII trial should provide some prospective information on this question; the rarity of specific genetic subtypes also calls for collaboration to determine which of the specific GIST genetic subtypes are most and least likely to benefit from 3 years of therapy.

Given the diminishing returns seen in patients treated with imatinib versus placebo in the recent SSG XVIII update, an affiliated commentary raised the concern that adjuvant imatinib is merely delaying recurrence rather than preventing it.[27] Interestingly, at least one of the authors of the commentary maintains some people on imatinib

**Table 1**
Gastrointestinal stromal tumor mutation status and in vitro and in vivo sensitivity to imatinib

| Gene | Exon | Mutation Type | Frequency Among Primary GIST (%)[13] | Sensitivity to Imatinib in Patients | Sensitivity to Imatinib In Vitro |
|---|---|---|---|---|---|
| KIT | 8 | | <1 | S | ? |
| | 9 | | 6 | I | S |
| | | AY502–503dup | | I | S |
| | 11 | | 66 | S | S |
| | | WK557–558del | | S | S |
| | | V560G | | S | S |
| | | L576P | | R | R |
| | 12 | | <1 | R | ? |
| | 13 | | 1 | S | S |
| | | K642E substitution | | S | S |
| | | D635K substitution | | | S |
| | 14 | | <1 | ? | ? |
| | 17 | | 1 | I? | S |
| | | N822 substitutions (eg, N822Y, N822K, N822H) | | I? | S |
| | 18 | | <1 | ? | ? |
| PDGFRA | 4 | | <1 | S | ? |
| | 10 | | <1 | ? | ? |
| | 12 | | 2 | S | S |
| | | SPDHE566–571R | | ? | S |
| | 14 | | <1 | ? | S |
| | | ER561–2 | | ? | S |
| | 18 | | 8 | I | I |
| | | D842V | 5–6 | R | R |
| | | N659K | | | S |
| | | D842Y | | | S |
| | | RD841–842KI | | | R |
| | | DI842–843IM | | | R |
| | | D846Y | | | S |
| | | N848K | | | S |
| | | Y849K | | | S |
| | | HDSN845–848P | | | S |
| KIT/PDGFRA mutation negative—includes all classes below | | | 16 | I | I? |
| SDH genes | — | Gene loss | | R | ? |
| NF1 | — | Gene loss | | R | I? |
| BRAF | 15 | V600E | | R | R |
| PIK3CA | Various | Possible resistance mutation | | R? | R? |

*Abbreviations:* ?, data uncertain, unavailable, or conflicting; I, intermediate; R, resistant; S, sensitive.
*Data from* Refs.[29–37]

indefinitely in the adjuvant setting. Should all high-risk patients be considered metastatic from the outset? Should imatinib be considered to be like hormonal therapy, expecting that longer exposure to drug (eg, 10 vs 5 years in trials of antiestrogens) will be associated with longer survival? Or will the imatinib-resistant clones known to pre-exist in primary tumor samples inevitably recur despite exposure to imatinib? It is hoped that molecular analyses from the SSG XVIII study will help with some of these questions in the near term, and the SSG XXII study may address some of these issues in the longer term.

It will be increasingly important to identify which patients stand any chance of improvement of the cure rate with imatinib. Perhaps larger and higher mitotic rate tumors are destined to recur and are thus not good candidates for adjuvant therapy, when giving imatinib in the relapse setting will suffice. Will it only be "Goldilocks" tumors with intermediate size and/or mutation rates be the only patients with sufficiently few micrometastases to benefit from imatinib? These and other questions will be of substantial interest in years to come, given the cost and symptom burden associated with imatinib.[28] By one very crude calculation at more than $100,000 per year for imatinib in the United States in 2016, for a 7% improvement in survival, more than $1.4 million must be spent to save one life.

Despite 15 years or more of experience with imatinib, it is still to be determined how best to use the drug in the adjuvant setting. The authors, among others, look forward to participating in research into both of these known unknowns and even the unknown unknowns that will better define the role of imatinib in the adjuvant as well as metastatic settings.

## REFERENCES

1. Hirota S, Isozaki K, Moriyama Y, et al. Gain-of-function mutations of c-kit in human gastrointestinal stromal tumors. Science 1998;279:577–80.

2. Wardelmann E, Merkelbach-Bruse S, Pauls K, et al. Polyclonal evolution of multiple secondary KIT mutations in gastrointestinal stromal tumors under treatment with imatinib mesylate. Clin Cancer Res 2006;12:1743–9.

3. Tuveson DA, Willis NA, Jacks T, et al. STI571 inactivation of the gastrointestinal stromal tumor c-KIT oncoprotein: biological and clinical implications. Oncogene 2001;20:5054–8.

4. Joensuu H, Roberts PJ, Sarlomo-Rikala M, et al. Effect of the tyrosine kinase inhibitor STI571 in a patient with a metastatic gastrointestinal stromal tumor. N Engl J Med 2001;344:1052–6.

5. van Oosterom AT, Judson I, Verweij J, et al. Safety and efficacy of imatinib (STI571) in metastatic gastrointestinal stromal tumours: a phase I study. Lancet 2001;358:1421–3.

6. Verweij J, Casali PG, Zalcberg J, et al. Progression-free survival in gastrointestinal stromal tumours with high-dose imatinib: randomised trial. Lancet 2004; 364:1127–34.

7. Demetri GD, van Oosterom AT, Garrett CR, et al. Efficacy and safety of sunitinib in patients with advanced gastrointestinal stromal tumour after failure of imatinib: a randomised controlled trial. Lancet 2006;368:1329–38.

8. Demetri GD, Reichardt P, Kang YK, et al. Efficacy and safety of regorafenib for advanced gastrointestinal stromal tumours after failure of imatinib and sunitinib (GRID): an international, multicentre, randomised, placebo-controlled, phase 3 trial. Lancet 2013;381:295–302.

9. Joensuu H, Eriksson M, Sundby Hall K, et al. One vs three years of adjuvant imatinib for operable gastrointestinal stromal tumor: a randomized trial. JAMA 2012; 307:1265–72.

10. Ng EH, Pollock RE, Munsell MF, et al. Prognostic factors influencing survival in gastrointestinal leiomyosarcomas. Implications for surgical management and staging. Ann Surg 1992;215:68–77.

11. DeMatteo RP, Lewis JJ, Leung D, et al. Two hundred gastrointestinal stromal tumors: recurrence patterns and prognostic factors for survival. Ann Surg 2000; 231:51–8.

12. Demetri GD, von Mehren M, Blanke CD, et al. Efficacy and safety of imatinib mesylate in advanced gastrointestinal stromal tumors. N Engl J Med 2002;347:472–80.

13. Joensuu H, Rutkowski P, Nishida T, et al. KIT and PDGFRA mutations and the risk of GI stromal tumor recurrence. J Clin Oncol 2015;33:634–42.

14. DeMatteo RP, Ballman KV, Antonescu CR, et al. Long-term results of adjuvant imatinib mesylate in localized, high-risk, primary gastrointestinal stromal tumor: ACOSOG Z9000 (Alliance) intergroup phase 2 trial. Ann Surg 2013;258:422–9.

15. Corless CL, Ballman KV, Antonescu CR, et al. Pathologic and molecular features correlate with long-term outcome after adjuvant therapy of resected primary GI stromal tumor: the ACOSOG Z9001 trial. J Clin Oncol 2014;32:1563–70.

16. Dematteo RP, Ballman KV, Antonescu CR, et al. Adjuvant imatinib mesylate after resection of localised, primary gastrointestinal stromal tumour: a randomised, double-blind, placebo-controlled trial. Lancet 2009;373:1097–104.

17. Casali PG, Le Cesne A, Poveda Velasco A, et al. Time to definitive failure to the first tyrosine kinase inhibitor in localized GI stromal tumors treated with imatinib as an adjuvant: a European Organisation for Research and Treatment of Cancer Soft Tissue and Bone Sarcoma Group Intergroup Randomized Trial in collaboration with the Australasian Gastro-Intestinal Trials Group, UNICANCER, French Sarcoma Group, Italian Sarcoma Group, and Spanish Group for research on sarcomas. J Clin Oncol 2015;33:4276–83.

18. Kang YK, Kang BW, Im SA, et al. Two-year adjuvant imatinib mesylate after complete resection of localized, high-risk GIST with KIT exon 11 mutation. Cancer Chemother Pharmacol 2013;71:43–51.

19. Joensuu H, Eriksson M, Sundby Hall K, et al. Adjuvant imatinib for high-risk GI stromal tumor: analysis of a randomized trial. J Clin Oncol 2016;34:244–50.

20. Wang D, Zhang Q, Blanke CD, et al. Phase II trial of neoadjuvant/adjuvant imatinib mesylate for advanced primary and metastatic/recurrent operable gastrointestinal stromal tumors: long-term follow-up results of Radiation Therapy Oncology Group 0132. Ann Surg Oncol 2012;19:1074–80.

21. Eisenberg BL, Harris J, Blanke CD, et al. Phase II trial of neoadjuvant/adjuvant imatinib mesylate (IM) for advanced primary and metastatic/recurrent operable gastrointestinal stromal tumor (GIST): early results of RTOG 0132/ACRIN 6665. J Surg Oncol 2009;99:42–7.

22. Jakob J, Mussi C, Ronellenfitsch U, et al. Gastrointestinal stromal tumor of the rectum: results of surgical and multimodality therapy in the era of imatinib. Ann Surg Oncol 2013;20:586–92.

23. Joensuu H, Reichardt P, Eriksson M, et al. Gastrointestinal stromal tumor: a method for optimizing the timing of CT scans in the follow-up of cancer patients. Radiology 2014;271:96–103.

24. von Mehren M, Randall RL, Benjamin RS, et al. NCCN Clinical Practice Guidelines in Oncology: Soft Tissue Sarcoma, (ed 02.2016). 2016. Available at: nccn.org. Accessed May 13, 2016.

25. Joensuu H, Martin-Broto J, Nishida T, et al. Follow-up strategies for patients with gastrointestinal stromal tumour treated with or without adjuvant imatinib after surgery. Eur J Cancer 2015;51:1611–7.

26. ESMO/European Sarcoma Network Working Group. Gastrointestinal stromal tumours: ESMO Clinical Practice Guidelines for diagnosis, treatment and follow-up. Ann Oncol 2014;25(Suppl 3):iii21–6.

27. Benjamin RS, Casali PG. Adjuvant imatinib for GI stromal tumors: when and for how long. J Clin Oncol 2016;34:215–8.

28. Sanon M, Taylor DC, Parthan A, et al. Cost-effectiveness of 3-years of adjuvant imatinib in gastrointestinal stromal tumors (GIST) in the United States. J Med Econ 2013;16:150–9.

29. Heinrich MC, Maki RG, Corless CL, et al. Primary and secondary kinase genotypes correlate with the biological and clinical activity of sunitinib in imatinib-resistant gastrointestinal stromal tumor. J Clin Oncol 2008;26:5352–9.

30. Lasota J, Felisiak-Golabek A, Wasag B, et al. Frequency and clinicopathologic profile of PIK3CA mutant GISTs: molecular genetic study of 529 cases. Mod Pathol 2016;29(3):275–82.

31. Debiec-Rychter M, Sciot R, Le Cesne A, et al. KIT mutations and dose selection for imatinib in patients with advanced gastrointestinal stromal tumours. Eur J Cancer 2006;42:1093–103.

32. Lasota J, Miettinen M. Clinical significance of oncogenic KIT and PDGFRA mutations in gastrointestinal stromal tumours. Histopathology 2008;53:245–66.

33. Maertens O, Prenen H, Debiec-Rychter M, et al. Molecular pathogenesis of multiple gastrointestinal stromal tumors in NF1 patients. Hum Mol Genet 2006;15:1015–23.

34. Cassier PA, Fumagalli E, Rutkowski P, et al. Outcome of patients with platelet-derived growth factor receptor alpha-mutated gastrointestinal stromal tumors in the tyrosine kinase inhibitor era. Clin Cancer Res 2012;18:4458–64.

35. Antonescu CR, Busam KJ, Francone TD, et al. L576P KIT mutation in anal melanomas correlates with KIT protein expression and is sensitive to specific kinase inhibition. Int J Cancer 2007;121:257–64.

36. Conca E, Negri T, Gronchi A, et al. Activate and resist: L576P-KIT in GIST. Mol Cancer Ther 2009;8:2491–5.

37. Janeway KA, Albritton KH, Van Den Abbeele AD, et al. Sunitinib treatment in pediatric patients with advanced GIST following failure of imatinib. Pediatr Blood Cancer 2009;52:767–71.

# Neuroendocrine Tumors

Ron Basuroy, MD, MBA, Raj Srirajaskanthan, MD, FRCP,
John K. Ramage, MD, FRCP*

## KEYWORDS

- Neuroendocrine • Tumor • Multimodal • Therapy • Carcinoid • Diagnostics

## KEY POINTS

- Neuroendocrine tumors are heterogenous in nature and increasing in incidence.
- Symptoms can develop from secreted bioactive substances or from the mass effect of the tumor.
- Anatomic and functional imaging modalities are helpful in staging disease and assessing tumor biology.
- A range of therapies is available that include surgical, liver directed, and systemic therapies.
- The treatment of neuroendocrine tumors can be multimodal over a patient's disease history.

## INTRODUCTION

Neuroendocrine tumors (NETs) of the gastrointestinal tract arise at many different sites, including the pancreas and small bowel, and are heterogeneous in nature with increasing incidence.[1] This review of gastroenteropancreatic (GEP) NETs discusses epidemiology, presentation, diagnosis, and management of primary and secondary sites of disease. Gastroenterologists have traditionally diagnosed and managed these tumors but now have a core role in multidisciplinary tumor board meetings on therapy decisions like surgery and systemic therapies. Significant advances have been made in managing these tumors with new diagnostics techniques and therapies. Many patients are now informed about their condition with information from Web sites and patient support groups with an expectation to access the whole array of diagnostic and therapeutic modalities.

NETs originate from neuroendocrine cells in the pancreatic islet and gastroenteric tissue. Small bowel (sb) and pancreatic (p) NETs have different clinical and genetic signatures and were previously considered to be largely benign in nature. The World Health Organization (WHO) 2010 nomenclature considers all NETs as malignant and classifies them by the cellular proliferation and degree of differentiation.[2] The use of NET rather

Neuroendocrine Tumour Unit, Institute of Liver Studies, Kings College Hospital, Denmark Hill, London SE5 9RS, UK
* Corresponding author. Department of Gastroenterology, Hampshire Hospitals NHS Trust, Basingstoke RG24 9NA.
E-mail address: John.Ramage@hhft.nhs.uk

Gastroenterol Clin N Am 45 (2016) 487–507
http://dx.doi.org/10.1016/j.gtc.2016.04.007
0889-8553/16/$ – see front matter Crown Copyright © 2016 Published by Elsevier Inc. All rights reserved.

than the historical "carcinoid" tumor is preferred and encouraged for describing gastro-intestinal and pNETs. Similarly, classification by primary tumor site rather than embryo-logic origin (foregut/midgut/hindgut) is the accepted nomenclature. The molecular biology of NETs is still poorly understood, but there are emerging data to suggest that profiling of genetic and molecular signatures may enhance tumor classification and identify potential targets that may be involved in tumor progression[3] (Table 1).

## Epidemiology

A key problem with NET epidemiology has been changes to classification systems and reliance on registries. International Classification of Diseases for Oncology-10 uses histopathological coding and has been used in most recent registries. It includes all the tumors that were previously classified as benign, which may be partly contributing to the increased incidence since 2000.[4] The largest registry is the Surveillance, Epide-miology, and End Results database that spans more than 5 decades and 15% of the US population from specific states.[5,6] There are national population studies that contribute to defining incidence in the United Kingdom, Norway, Sweden, Ireland, Netherlands, Denmark, and Austria.[7–12] NETs may now be the most common small bowel tumor (37.4%), ahead of adenocarcinoma (36.9%), lymphomas (17.3%), and stromal tumors (8.4%).[13]

There are reported ethnic differences with African Americans having the highest NET incidence at 6.5 per 100,000 persons.[6,14] The overall incidence of NETs in Caucasians in the United States and Norway is 4.44 and 3.24 per 100,000 persons, respectively.[10] The rectum is the commonest site in the United States and Far East, with lung NETs the commonest site in Caucasian US patients.[15,16] The incidence of NETS of the appendix, cecum, and pancreas almost doubled between 1975 and 2005, but these tumors are only a fraction of NETs diagnosed, around 0.1 to 0.2 cases per 100,000 persons. Historical autopsy studies in Sweden described an incidence of 8.4 per 100,000 with a significant number of NET tumors that were not diagnosed antemortem.[17] The prevalence of NET is proportionally much greater than the inci-dence because of improved survival when compared with other common cancers like gastric and pancreatic adenocarcinomas.[18] Whatever the precise incidence of NETs, it appears that the number of patients presenting with these tumors has been steadily increasing.

## Genetics

GEP-NETs may be associated with familial endocrine cancer syndromes, such as pNETs with multiple endocrine neoplasia type 1 (MEN1) and less commonly with von Hippel-Lindau and tuberous sclerosis. The incidence of MEN1 in GEP NETs varies

**Table 1**
**World Health Organization classification of neuroendocrine tumors**

| WHO (2010) and ENETS Nomenclature | Grade | Mitotic Count | Ki-67 Index (%) | Cell Type |
|---|---|---|---|---|
| NET | G1 | <2 mitoses/10 HPF | ≤2 | — |
| NET | G2 | 2–20 mitoses/10 HPF | 3–20 | — |
| Neuroendocrine carcinoma (NEC) | G3 | >20 mitoses/10 HPF | >20 | Large vs small cell |

*Abbreviation:* ENETS, European Neuroendocrine Tumor Society.
*From* Bosman F. WHO classification of tumours of the digestive system. Lyon (France): IARC Press; 2010; with permission.

from rare in gastrointestinal (GI) NET, to 5% in insulinomas, and 25% to 30% in gastrinomas.[19,20] The diagnosis of MEN1 can now be confirmed by testing for the presence of the MENIN gene mutation. Mutations involving the succinate dehydrogenase subunit D, usually associated with paragangliomas and pheochromocytomas can be associated with sbNETs.[21]

There are sb and colon "NET families" (non-MEN1) described in which more than one family member has been diagnosed with an NET. Standardized incidence rates of 4.35 for small intestinal and 4.65 for colon NETs occur in offspring of parents affected by NETs. Candidate genes for these findings have been proposed.[22,23]

There has been recent interest in somatic mutations occurring in these tumors.[3] Jiao and colleagues[3] sequenced tissue from pNET and found an excess of mutations in the menin, DAXX, ATRXX, and mTOR genes. Differences in survival related to the presence of these genes have been debated, but the work may lead to personalized medicine based on genetics results.[24]

## CLINICAL PRESENTATIONS OF GASTROENTEROPANCREATIC NEUROENDOCRINE TUMORS

NETs are described in the pancreas and all sites of the gastrointestinal tract. The behavior of GEP-NETs does differ by primary site with symptoms varying from the incidental diagnosis through to obstructive mass effect and symptomatic syndromes from the secretion of bioactive agents. There may be a significant delay between onset of symptoms and diagnosis.[25] Diarrhea and flushing are known specific symptoms, but frequently fatigue is the worst symptom with depression also common. Quality-of-life (QoL) research in GEP-NETs is a comparatively new field, with a disease-specific QoL questionnaire, the QLQ-GINET21, and the Norfolk NET questionnaire being used in trials for GI NET.[26] Symptomatic patients frequently have liver metastases at diagnosis. The liver lesions are highly vascular and can be "functionally" active secreting vasoactive substances or hormones that can cause systemic symptoms. The 4 commonest GEP-NET primary sites are discussed later (**Table 2**).

### Small Bowel

sbNETs are equal to rectal tumors in being the next most common primary site of all NETs (after lung) with an incidence of 17.2%.[18,27] The most common site is the last

**Table 2**
**Neuroendocrine tumor symptom duration with ages at diagnosis and onset from a UK patient questionnaire**

| Type of NET | No. | Mean Age at Diagnosis | Mean Duration 1st Symptom (Range, mo) | Mean Age at 1st Symptom (y) | Age Over 50 at 1st Symptom (%) |
|---|---|---|---|---|---|
| Appendix | 14 | 44.2 | 46.8 (2–180) | 41.7 | 29 |
| Lung | 51 | 50.7 | 67.7 (1.5–360) | 46.2 | 54 |
| Pancreas | 64 | 49.2 | 39.1 (0–240) | 46.6 | 42 |
| Small bowel | 99 | 55.2 | 60.1 (0–300) | 50.8 | 69 |
| Stomach/gastric | 14 | 55.1 | 38.5 (1–144) | 53.0 | 71 |
| Unknown Primary | 33 | 52.9 | 43.4 (1.5–204) | 50.4 | 55 |
| Grand total | 275 | 52.1 | 53.3 (0–360) | 48.6 | 56 |

*From* Basuroy R, Bouvier C, Sissons M, et al. The symptoms experienced by small bowel and pancreatic NET patients prior to diagnosis do not meet the criteria for a functional diarrhoea (IBS-D) diagnosis. UKI NETS 13th National Conference. London, December 7, 2015; with permission.

60 cm of distal ileum with a quarter being multifocal tumors.[28] Common symptoms are of abdominal pain as well as intermitted bowel obstruction that can result from the mechanical effect of the primary tumor, or from mesenteric lymph node involvement, secondary desmoplasia, and bowel ischemia from vessel involvement.[29,30] sbNETs can cause the classical carcinoid syndrome of diarrhea, flushing, palpitations, and bronchospasm, which develop in the context of serotonin-secreting liver metastases. Carcinoid heart disease can develop from fibrosis of the tricuspid and pulmonary valves, leading to right heart failure in patients with carcinoid syndrome and elevated serotonin.[31,32] Prolonged serotonin production in carcinoid syndrome may lead to nicotinamide deficiency, causing lacrimation, rhinorrhea, and diarrhea.

### Rectum

The incidence of rectal NETs has increased rapidly to 17% of all NETs and now equals that of sbNETs in recent years.[5,6,14] Most patients are asymptomatic with over half of all rectal NETs diagnosed incidentally at endoscopy.[33] Rectal NETs have the best overall survival of GEP-NETs, with almost 90% less than 1 cm and localized to the submucosal.[34]

### Stomach

The incidence of gastric NETs has increased to 6.0% of all NETs between 2000 and 2007.[35,36] Gastric NETs are invariably diagnosed at endoscopy and arise from enterochromaffin-like cells involved in the regulation of gastric acid production.[37] Three subtypes are described with type 1 and type 2 developing in the presence of hypergastrinemia, and type 3 occurring independently of gastrin. Type 1 gastric NETs develop from secondary hypergastrinemia stimulation from achlorhydria environments like chronic atrophic gastritis. Type 2 gastric NETs develop from autonomous hypergastrinemia stimulation from a gastrinoma that can cause marked acid secretion and peptic ulceration. Histamine secretion can occur in gastric NETs causing allergic-type symptoms.

### Pancreas

The incidence of pNETs is approximately 6% of all NETs, with a less rapid increase when compared with rectal and gastric NETs incidences that are more directly influenced by increased endoscopy.[18] Almost half of pNETs are functional with symptoms that result from bioactive secretion as outlined in later discussion. The value of classifying tumors by specific hormone output has been challenged, although it is still common practice.[38] Nonfunctional pNETs are often incidental findings on cross-sectional imaging, but a proportion of patients present with symptoms from mass effect, such as biliary obstruction, or from metastatic disease[39] (**Table 3**).

**Table 3**
**Neuroendocrine tumors that secrete bioactive substances**

| Tumor Type | Symptoms |
| --- | --- |
| Insulinoma | Dizziness, irritability, sweating, fits, coma, response to food |
| Gastrinoma | Small bowel perforation, duodenal ulceration with bleeding, diarrhea responding to PPI therapy |
| Glucagonoma | Diabetes, migratory rash, diarrhea, stomatitis |
| VIPoma | Severe diarrhea, weight loss, hypokalemia |
| Somatostinoma | Gall stones, weight loss, diarrhea, steatorrhea, diabetes |
| PPoma | Usually no specific symptoms; weight gain and constipation can occur |

## DIAGNOSTIC MODALITIES

Anatomic imaging modalities, such as computed tomography (CT) and MRI, characterize the extent of NET disease to assist with staging and planning therapy.[40] In particular, CT provides an anatomic map for both curative and debulking cytoreductive surgical resections. Functional imaging modalities, like octreotide scintigraphy and PET-CT, provide evidence of biological behavior that, as discussed later in the review, indicate the role for the specific medical therapies in disease management.

### Anatomic Imaging

CT is the dominant anatomic imaging modality for NETs, which exhibit avid early enhancement (pNETs in particular) on biphasic or triphasic contrast-enhanced CT. Unenhanced scans can demonstrate an isodense lesion with calcification in 20% of pNETs in contrast to the uncalcified appearances of pancreatic adenocarcinomas.[41] pNETs typically show homogenous avid arterial enhancement with contrast. Nonfunctional pNETs are typically larger than functional pNETs and can be heterogenous lesions with necrosis and cystic degeneration as well as can cause mass effect on surrounding structures like the biliary system.

sbNETs typically cause a marked desmoplastic reaction in the mesentery with fat changes, tethering, and stranding that are easily discernible on CT. In addition, nodal metastases to the root of the mesentery can encase vessels like the superior mesenteric vein (SMV) and superior mesenteric artery (SMA) with consequent radiological signs of bowel ischemia. Metastatic disease to the liver enhances in a similar pattern to the primary NET. The hepatic arterial phase is useful in identifying liver metastases.[42] The sensitivity of CT in detecting primary, regional, and metastatic disease increases with lesion size.

MRI is a useful imaging modality in NETs given the burden of ionizing radiation exposure from diagnosis through to surveillance in patients. pNETs typically exhibit T2-weighted (T2W) hyperintensity and T1-weighted (T1W) hypointensity with moderate but diffuse contrast enhancement.[43,44] Two-thirds of sbNETs can be identified on MRI and are more easily discernible on postgadolinium contrast T1W fat-suppressed images.[45] MRI can help characterize liver metastases when CT is equivocal or when the background liver is steatotic. Lesions are more easily identified on T2W and hepatic arterial phase T1W fat-suppressed imaging.[46] Diffusion-weighted imaging is useful in characterizing NETs, particularly pNETs and hepatic metastases, as well as assessing response to liver directed therapy[47–49] (**Figs. 1** and **2**).

### Functional Imaging

Somatostatin receptors (SSTR) are differentially expressed in NETs with most GEP-NETs expressing the subtype SSTR2.[50,51] Functional imaging modalities assess for SSTR2 expression and can provide additional staging and prognostic information beyond cross-sectional modalities. Importantly, patients with lesions that are SSTR2-avid can benefit from specific therapeutic options that are discussed later.[52] [111]Indium-octreotide scintigraphy (OctreoScan) and PET-CT with [68]Ga-DOTATATE are useful modalities for assessing for avid disease in patients with low-grade (G1 or G2) and well-differentiated GEP-NETs. [68]Ga-DOTATATE PET has a higher sensitivity and specificity than [111]Indium-octreotide scintigraphy.[53] High-grade (G3) and poorly differentiated NETs have lower expression of SSTR and are consequently poorly avid. However, these tumor lesions are metabolically more active and take up the glucose analogue on PET with fludeoxyglucose F 18 imaging[54] (**Figs. 3** and **4**).

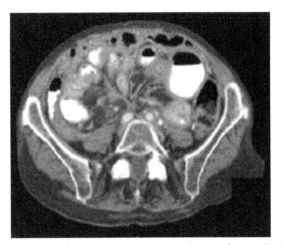

**Fig. 1.** CT demonstrating the characteristic mesenteric changes from a sbNET with tethering as well as thick-walled bowel.

## MARKERS OF NEUROENDOCRINE TUMORS DISEASE

Circulating and tissue markers of NET disease can be used to assess for disease, prognosis, treatment response, and recurrence.[55] Existing markers may be general, like chromogranin A (CgA) and serotonin, or specific to subtypes of NETs like gastrin and insulin. More novel markers, like mRNA transcript panels and circulating tumor cells, are likely to have a role in the future.[56–59]

### Chromogranin A

CgA is a soluble protein stored and secreted by NETs and has the most clinical utility for diagnosis, prognosis and treatment response.[60–62] A meta-analysis has shown that CgA has high sensitivity (73%) and specificity (95%) for the diagnosis of NETs.[63] The sensitivity of CgA varies according to the primary site, with higher sensitivity for gastrinomas (100%) and gastric NETs (95%) but lower sensitivity for pancreatic (70%) NETs. CgA is of greater clinical utility in G1 and G2 NETs. An elevated CgA is predictive

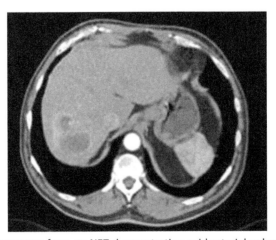

**Fig. 2.** Hepatic metastases from an NET demonstrating avid arterial enhancement.

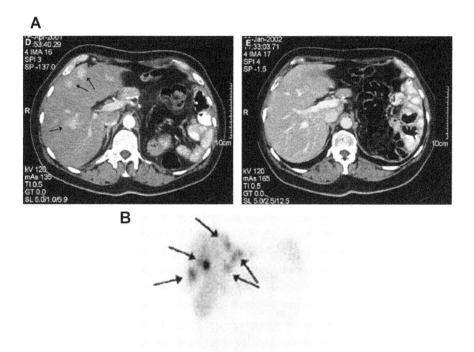

**Fig. 3.** CT scan (*A*) and Octreoscan (*B*) depicting neuroendocrine hepatic metastases (*arrows*), which are avid on functional imaging assessment.

of shorter survival in small bowel and pNETs. The CgA assay can be falsely elevated by other non-NET factors like proton pump inhibitors (PPI) use and renal impairment.

### Serotonin and 5-Hydroxyindoleacetic Acid

Carcinoid syndrome develops from the secretion of 5-hydroxytryptamine (5-HT or serotonin) and other vasoactive peptides.[64] The secreted products from sbNETs can cause a local mesenteric desmoplastic reaction as well as distant fibrosis of the cardiac valves resulting in carcinoid heart disease. 5-HT secretion can be measured directly in serum and platelet assays as well as indirectly from its metabolite

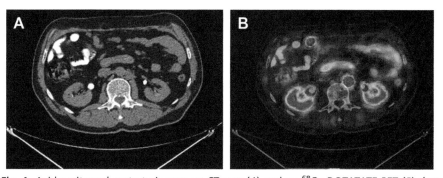

**Fig. 4.** Avid peritoneal metastasis seen on CT scan (*A*) and on [68]Ga-DOTATATE PET (*B*) that was not identified on Octreoscan.

5-hydroxyindoleacetic acid in the urine. Elevated levels correlate with the likelihood of carcinoid heart disease and liver metastases.

## MANAGEMENT

Therapies for GEP-NETs are ideally aimed at a cure but also focus on symptom control and antiproliferative effects. The management of NETs requires the use of several different therapies including surgery, biotherapy, chemotherapy, peptide receptor radionuclide therapy (PRRT), and tumor embolization. A multidisciplinary approach is advocated given the multimodal approach to managing NET patients.[1] Patients with advanced disease or recurrence may require several different therapies over their disease therapy, while others may have a more indolent disease and minimal symptoms that are well controlled for years.

### Surgery for Primary Neuroendocrine Tumors

Surgery remains the only method for cure and should be considered in all patients if technically feasible. Patients with localized GEP-NET tumors should be offered curative surgical resection of the primary lesion. The surgical management should be individualized for each patient given oncologic and technical considerations as well as comorbidities.

Nonrandomized studies have demonstrated a survival benefit for pNET patients from surgery.[65] Curative surgery in patients with metastatic pNETs offers a survival benefit following resections of primary and metastatic disease.[66] The role of primary resection in the context of unresectable metastatic disease is less clear but there may be some benefit at meta-analysis of nonrandomized studies.[66]

The resection of a primary sbNET and nodal mesenteric mass improves survival.[67,68] Furthermore, many retrospective studies and meta-analyses have suggested benefit from resecting the primary sbNET in the context of unresectable metastatic disease.[69] Benefit is thought to be due to the reduction in risk of complications, such as small bowel obstruction due to tumor mass effect. Similarly, resection of both primary sbNET and hepatic metastases has an acceptable mortality and morbidity with excellent long-term survival rates.[67]

### Liver-directed Therapies

The size, number, and distribution of liver metastases are important factors that affect survival and treatment strategies.[70,71] Solitary liver metastases can be resected with curative intent and can have 5-year survivals of 100%. Debulking surgery for liver disease should be considered a palliative option in patients with symptoms related to carcinoid syndrome refractory to medical therapy or in whom there is evidence of clinical or radiologic progression of disease. Debulking of greater than 90% of the hepatic tumor burden may lead to longer survival as well as symptom control.[72,73] However, a Cochrane Review to assess the role of debulking surgery or cytoreductive surgery was equivocal due to the lack of high-quality data.[74,75]

#### Locoablative therapy for hepatic metastases
Several interventional radiology and surgical techniques are available for ablation of liver metastases. The methods available include radiofrequency ablation, microwave ablation, cryotherapy, and irreversible electroporation. These methods can be performed percutaneously, laparoscopically, or at open surgery. Radiofrequency ablation series describe a 5-year overall survival of 53% with a local hepatic recurrence rate of 22% and new hepatic lesions in 63% of patients.[76,77] There are no data to suggest an

improvement in overall survival with ablative therapies primarily used for symptom control from reduced hormone secretion.

### Hepatic artery embolization

Embolization of the liver can result in necrosis of metastatic tumor tissue resulting in decreased hormonal secretion. Hepatic artery embolization (HAE) can offer good tumor control, although there are limited data on improvements in overall survival.[78] Symptomatic response is seen in 40% to 80% of cases with a biochemical response for hepatic embolization of 7% to 75% and 12% to 75% for hepatic chemoembolization.[78,79] A study by Gupta and colleagues[78] demonstrated no additional benefit of chemotherapy to transcatheter arterial embolization in metastatic small bowel tumors. Contraindications to performing HAE include portal vein thrombosis, liver failure, and biliary reconstruction as well as a patient's poor performance status. Postembolization complications include ileus, portal vein thrombosis, hepatic abscess, hepatic fistula, encephalopathy, and renal insufficiency (**Table 4**).

### Selective internal radiation therapy

Hepatic embolization with Yttrium-90 ($^{90}$Y) selective internal radiation therapy (SIRT) has been used for over a decade with a small number of studies in NET patients.[88–91] A study by Kennedy and colleagues[89] in 148 patients with unresectable NET liver metastases demonstrated stable disease in 22.7%, partial response in 60.5%, and complete response in 2.7%. $^{90}$Y microspheres have been better tolerated than chemoembolization in these studies. A recent single-center retrospective series of 40 patients reported an objective tumor response and disease control rates of 54% and 94%, respectively, with a mean overall survival from the first SIRT of 34.8 months.[92]

## Medical Therapies for Neuroendocrine Tumors

Several therapy options are available for treating NET patients with advanced or progressive disease with significant survival benefit. An approach is to tailor therapy on the basis of tumor biology, predominantly from primary site, grade, and functional imaging results.

### Somatostatin analogues

Somatostatin analogues (SSA) are prescribed on the basis of SSTR expression, most commonly ascertained by tumor avidity from functional imaging assessment. Octreotide was the first synthetic analogue of somatostatin developed and reduces hormonal secretion.[93] The original preparation has a short half-life requiring intravenous or 3-times-daily subcutaneous dosing regimen to maintain steady levels.[94] Long-acting preparations (28 days) have been developed, but short-acting analogues are useful for breakthrough symptoms and in the perioperative period.[95–97]

Moreover, long-acting analogues (LAR) have been demonstrated to have an antiproliferative effect. A randomized placebo-controlled prospective study in patients with metastatic sbNETs demonstrated that long-acting octreotide inhibited tumor growth and delayed time to progression.[98] A further study in GEP-NETs (CLARINET) using lanreotide confirmed the antiproliferative effects of SSAs with significantly prolonged progression-free survival (PFS; median not reached vs median of 18.0 months, $P<.001$).[99]

Tolerance to SSAs is a recognized phenomenon, and there is a need for new biotherapy agents. Pasireotide, a new multiligand SSA, has completed a phase III study to assess control of functional symptoms in patients with metastatic NET. In this study, pasireotide LAR was compared with octreotide LAR in patients with

**Table 4**
Response rates to hepatic embolization and chemoembolization

| Study | Type of NET | HACE or HAE | No. of Patients | Clinical Response (%) | Biochemical Response (%) | Radiological Response (%) |
|---|---|---|---|---|---|---|
| Rusniewski et al,[80] 1993 | Small bowel | HACE | 24 | 73 | 57 | 33 |
| Therasse et al,[81] 1993 | Small bowel | HACE | 23 | 100 | 91 | 35 |
| Clouse et al,[82] 1994 | Small bowel | HACE | 14 | 90 | 69 | 78 |
| Diaco et al,[83] 1995 | Small bowel | HACE | 10 | 100 | — | 60 |
| Roche et al,[84] 2003 | Small bowel | HACE | 14 | 70 | 75 | 86 |
| Kim et al,[85] 1999 | Pancreatic | HACE | 14 | — | 90 | 50 |
| | Small bowel | | 16 | — | 75 | 25 |
| Drougas et al,[86] 1998 | Small bowel | HACE | 14 | 66 | 100 | — |
| Gupta et al,[78] 2005 | Small bowel | HAE or HACE | 69 | — | — | 67 |
| | Pancreatic | | 54 | | | 35 |
| Marrache et al,[87] 2007 | Small bowel | HACE | 48 | 91 | 65 | 37 |
| | Pancreatic | | 19 | | | |

Biochemical response is greater than 50% reduction in tumor markers CgA. Radiological response is reduction in tumor volume greater than 50% using cross-sectional imaging.

*Abbreviations:* HACE, hepatic artery chemoembolization; HAE, hepatic artery embolization.

uncontrolled NET symptoms and did not demonstrate any significant improvement in symptoms.[100] However, a median investigator-assessed PFS of 11.8 months for pasireotide (vs 6.8 months for octreotide) was observed (hazard ratio = 0.46; $P$ = .045).

### Interferon-$\alpha$

Interferon therapy has been used since 1982 for symptom control with 50% to 60% of carcinoid syndrome patients experiencing a reduction in flushing and diarrhea.[94] Significant biochemical responses are reported in 40% to 50% of cases. Its mechanism of action is unclear, although it is thought to act through antisecretory and immunomodulatory functions.

### Chemotherapy

Chemotherapy has been widely used as first-line therapy for unresectable poorly differentiated NETs and well-differentiated pNETs. The results from different pNET chemotherapy regimens are variable. The response rates demonstrated by Moertel nearly 40 years ago have been difficult to replicate in recent studies.[101] Most chemotherapy trials have been single-center retrospective series. However, the multicenter randomized prospective study NET-01 study reported recently on the addition of cisplatin to capecitabine and streptozocin (STZ) in GEP-NETs patients. It demonstrated no benefit of adding cisplatin to a capecitabine and STZ regimen. The disease control rate was 80% with the medical PFS of 10.2 months.[102] STZ-based combinations are an accepted first-line chemotherapy regimen for well-differentiated G1 or G2 pNETs.

In well-differentiated pNETs, there is also evidence emerging regarding the use of Temozolomide, either as monotherapy or in combination with capecitabine.[103] A retrospective study of temozolomide combined with capecitabine in 30 chemotherapy-naive patients demonstrated an objective radiographic response rate of 70% and a median PFS of 18 months.[104] In contrast, the overall response rate for sbNETs to a range of chemotherapy agents is less than 30%[105–108] (**Table 5**).

### Peptide receptor radionuclide therapy

PRRT is a systemic therapy using radiolabeled SSAs that bind to SSTR expressed on GEP-NETs and are internalized causing radiation-induced cell death. PRRT has been in use in Europe since the early 1990s but has not been approved by the US Food and Drug Administration in the United States. There is a large amount of data from single centers across Europe and only a single phase 3 randomized controlled trial (RCT) that has recently reported interim results.[116,117]

The two commonly used radionuclide therapies are yttrium Y-90-DOTA-octreotate and lutetium Lu-177-DOTA-octreotate, which both have similar efficacies.[118,119] Across all studies, symptomatic improvement has been reported in 60% to 80% of cases. Partial tumor response of greater than 50% tumor load is seen in 9% to 33% of patients, whereas stable disease is reported in approximately two-thirds of cases. The first phase 3 randomized control study (NETTER-1) for Lutetium DOTATATE therapy in sbNETs patients with carcinoid syndrome recently reported and demonstrated an improved survival benefit when compared with octreotide LAR 60 mg 4 weekly.[117] The objective response rate was 19% in the NETTER-1 study, although radiological response rates were lower than those reported in retrospective studies.

The main adverse effect with radiopeptide receptor therapy is due to the cumulative effect of bone marrow suppression, often seen after 3 doses. Other side effects include fatigue, tiredness, nausea, and, occasionally, liver failure. Long-term renal impairment can occur and is a key contraindication for therapy in patients. Bodei

**Table 5**
Response rates from chemotherapy in well and poorly differentiated neuroendocrine tumors

| Study | Regimen | No. of Patients | Objective Response (%) | Response Duration | Median Survival (mo) |
|---|---|---|---|---|---|
| Well-differentiated GEP NETs | | | | | |
| Moertel & Hanley,[108] 1979 | STZ + cyclophosphamide | 42 | 33 | 17 | 28.4 small bowel |
| | STZ + 5-FU | 47 | 26 | 17 | 28.4 pancreas |
| Moertel et al,[106] 1992 | Dox + STZ | 36 | 69 | 20 | 26 |
| | STZ + 5-FU | 33 | 45 | 6.9 | 18 |
| Eriksson et al,[107] 1990 | Dox + STZ | 25 | 24 | 22 | — |
| | STZ + 5-FU | 19 | 11 | | |
| Sun et al,[109] 2005 | Dox + 5-FU | 85 | 15.9 | 4.5 | — |
| | STZ + 5-FU | 78 | 16 | 5.3 | |
| Kulke et al,[110] 2006 | Irinotecan + cisplatin | 18 | 78 (only stable disease) | 4.5 | 11.4 |
| Kulke et al,[105] 2004 | Gemcitabine | 18 | 65 (only stable disease) | 8.3 | 11.5 |
| Rivera & Ajani,[111] 1998 | Dox + STZ + 5-FU | 12 | 55 | 15 | 21 |
| Kulke et al,[112] 2006 | Thalidomide + temozolomide | 29 | 25 | 13.5 | — |
| Poorly differentiated GEP NETs | | | | | |
| Moertel et al,[113] 1991 | Etoposide + cisplatin | 18 | 67 | 8 | 19 |
| Mitry et al,[114] 1999 | Etoposide + cisplatin | 41 | 42 | 9 | 15 |
| Mani et al,[115] 2008 | Irinotecan + cisplatin | 20 | 58 | 4 | — |

**Table 6**
**Response rates for peptide receptor therapy in neuroendocrine tumors**

| Authors | No. | Response (%) | | | | |
|---|---|---|---|---|---|---|
| | | CR | PR | MR | SD | PD |
| [90]Y-DOTATOC | | | | | | |
| Otte et al,[128] 1999 | 29 | 0 | 2 (7) | 4 (14) | 20 (69) | 3 (10) |
| Waldherre et al,[129] 2002 | 39 | 2 (55) | 7 (18) | n/a | 27 (69) | 3 (8) |
| Valkema et al,[130] 2006 | 52 | 0 | 5 (10) | 7 (13) | 29 (56) | 14 (26) |
| [90]Y-DOTATATE | | | | | | |
| Baum et al,[118] 2005 | 75 | 0 | 28 (37) | n/a | 39 (52) | 8 (11) |
| Lu[177]- DOTATATE | | | | | | |
| Kwekkeboom et al,[116] 2008 | 310 | 5 (2) | 96 (28) | 51 (16) | 107 (35) | 61 (20) |

Criteria for response used WHO criteria.
*Abbreviations:* CR, complete response; MR, minor response; n/a, not applicable; No., number of cases; PD, progressive disease; PR, partial response; SD, stable disease.

and colleagues[120] reported a decrease in creatinine clearance of between 5% and 10% in 20 of 23 patients treated with [90]Y at 1-year after therapy.

Some NETs have uptake of metaiodobenzylguanidine (MIBG), and therefore, radio-labeling MIBG is an alternative PRRT for targeted therapy. Since the first reports in 1994 of [131]I-MIBG therapy in NETs, many studies have been published showing variable response radiological response rates, with symptom response between 60% and 80%, with median duration of action between 6 and 24 months.[121–126] Treatment is well tolerated, and toxicity is often limited usually to temporary myelosuppression. Long-term follow-up data have demonstrated safety and efficacy[127] (**Table 6**).

### Everolimus

Everolimus is a mammalian target of rapamycin (mTOR) inhibitor that targets the serine-threonine kinase that stimulates cell growth, proliferation, and angiogenesis.[131] The RADIANT 3 study was the pivotal study that demonstrated a significantly longer PFS compared with placebo in patients with pNETs (11.0 vs 4.6 months; $P<.001$).[132] This treatment is licensed for use with well- or moderately differentiated pNETs and is generally well tolerated with common side effects including mucositis and fatigue. Recently, the RADIANT-4 study compared Everolimus alone or in combination with sandostatin LAR in patients with progressive unresectable pulmonary or sbNETs.[133] The results demonstrate an increase in PFS of 11 months when compared with sandostatin LAR supportive care alone.

### Sunitinib

Sunitinib is an inhibitor of multiple tyrosine kinase receptors, including platelet-derived growth factor receptor, vascular endothelial growth factor receptor, KIT, and RET. A phase III RCT demonstrated an increased PFS in patients with progressive pNETs compared with placebo (11.4 vs 5.5 months; $P<.001$).[134] This drug is licensed for use in well- to moderately differentiated pNETs.

### SUMMARY

- NETs are increasing in incidence, have a high prevalence, and are heterogenous in nature.
- Symptoms can be missed, resulting in late diagnosis.

- Pathologic classification (grading and staging) is complex but key to understanding tumor behavior.
- Recent advances in genetics may lead to personalized therapies.
- Imaging should include anatomic cross-sectional as well as functional methods. More sensitive modalities have developed in the last 10 years.
- Treatment methods are diverse, requiring initial assessment for surgery, followed by locoregional therapies (often to the liver), and then, if needed, systemic therapy, including PRRT, biological therapy, and chemotherapy.
- The field is advancing rapidly, and patients are best assessed in larger centers where all possible diagnostics and therapies are available.

## REFERENCES

1. Ramage JK, Ahmed A, Ardill J, et al. Guidelines for the management of gastroenteropancreatic neuroendocrine (including carcinoid) tumours (NETs). Gut 2012;61(1):6–32.
2. Bosman F. WHO classification of tumours of the digestive system. Lyon (France): IARC Press; 2010.
3. Jiao Y, Shi C, Edil BH, et al. DAXX/ATRX, MEN1, and mTOR pathway genes are frequently altered in pancreatic neuroendocrine tumors. Science 2011; 331(6021):1199–203.
4. World Health Organization. International classification of diseases for oncology. 3rd edition. Geneva (United Kingdom): World Health Organization; 2000.
5. Tsikitis VL, Wertheim BC, Guerrero MA. Trends of incidence and survival of gastrointestinal neuroendocrine tumors in the United States: a SEER analysis. J Cancer 2012;3:292–302.
6. Modlin IM, Lye KD, Kidd M. A 5-decade analysis of 13,715 carcinoid tumors. Cancer 2003;97(4):934–59.
7. Niederle MB, Hackl M, Kaserer K, et al. Gastroenteropancreatic neuroendocrine tumours: the current incidence and staging based on the WHO and European Neuroendocrine Tumour Society classification: an analysis based on prospectively collected parameters. Endocr Relat Cancer 2010;17(4):909–18.
8. Ito T, Sasano H, Tanaka M, et al. Epidemiological study of gastroenteropancreatic neuroendocrine tumors in Japan. J Gastroenterol 2010;45(2):234–43.
9. Ellis L, Shale MJ, Coleman MP. Carcinoid tumors of the gastrointestinal tract: trends in incidence in England since 1971. Am J Gastroenterol 2010;105(12): 2563–9.
10. Hauso O, Gustafsson BI, Kidd M, et al. Neuroendocrine tumor epidemiology: contrasting Norway and North America. Cancer 2008;113(10):2655–64.
11. Hemminki K, Li X. Incidence trends and risk factors of carcinoid tumors: a nationwide epidemiologic study from Sweden. Cancer 2001;92(8):2204–10.
12. Quaedvlieg PF, Visser O, Lamers CB, et al. Epidemiology and survival in patients with carcinoid disease in The Netherlands. An epidemiological study with 2391 patients. Ann Oncol 2001;12(9):1295–300.
13. Bilimoria KY, Bentrem DJ, Wayne JD, et al. Small bowel cancer in the United States: changes in epidemiology, treatment, and survival over the last 20 years. Ann Surg 2009;249(1):63–71.
14. Taghavi S, Jayarajan SN, Powers BD, et al. Examining rectal carcinoids in the era of screening colonoscopy: a surveillance, epidemiology, and end results analysis. Dis Colon Rectum 2013;56(8):952–9.

15. Konishi T, Watanabe T, Muto T, et al. Site distribution of gastrointestinal carcinoids differs between races. Gut 2006;55(7):1051–2.
16. Kotake K, Honjo S, Sugihara K, et al. Changes in colorectal cancer during a 20-year period: an extended report from the multi-institutional registry of large bowel cancer. Dis Colon Rectum 2003;46(Suppl 10):S32–43.
17. Berge T, Linell F. Carcinoid tumours. Frequency in a defined population during a 12-year period. Acta Pathol Microbiol Scand A 1976;84(4):322–30.
18. Yao JC, Hassan M, Phan A, et al. One hundred years after "carcinoid": epidemiology of and prognostic factors for neuroendocrine tumors in 35,825 cases in the United States. J Clin Oncol 2008;26(18):3063–72.
19. Debas HT, Mulvihill SJ. Neuroendocrine gut neoplasms. Important lessons from uncommon tumors. Arch Surg 1994;129(9):965–71 [discussion: 971–2].
20. Carroll RW. Multiple endocrine neoplasia type 1 (MEN1). Asia Pac J Clin Oncol 2013;9(4):297–309.
21. Kytola S, Nord B, Elder EE, et al. Alterations of the SDHD gene locus in midgut carcinoids, Merkel cell carcinomas, pheochromocytomas, and abdominal paragangliomas. Genes Chromosomes Cancer 2002;34(3):325–32.
22. Nilsson O. Profiling of ileal carcinoids. Neuroendocrinology 2013;97(1):7–18.
23. Banck MS, Kanwar R, Kulkarni AA, et al. The genomic landscape of small intestine neuroendocrine tumors. J Clin Invest 2013;123(6):2502–8.
24. Marinoni I, Kurrer AS, Vassella E, et al. Loss of DAXX and ATRX are associated with chromosome instability and reduced survival of patients with pancreatic neuroendocrine tumors. Gastroenterology 2014;146(2):453–60.e5.
25. Modlin IM, Kidd M, Latich I, et al. Current status of gastrointestinal carcinoids. Gastroenterology 2005;128(6):1717–51.
26. Yadegarfar G, Friend L, Jones L, et al. Validation of the EORTC QLQ-GINET21 questionnaire for assessing quality of life of patients with gastrointestinal neuroendocrine tumours. Br J Cancer 2013;108(2):301–10.
27. Strosberg J. Neuroendocrine tumours of the small intestine. Best Pract Res Clin Gastroenterol 2012;26(6):755–73.
28. Moertel CG. Karnofsky Memorial Lecture. An odyssey in the land of small tumors. J Clin Oncol 1987;5(10):1502–22.
29. Eckhauser FE, Argenta LC, Strodel WE, et al. Mesenteric angiopathy, intestinal gangrene, and midgut carcinoids. Surgery 1981;90(4):720–8.
30. Kulke MH, Mayer RJ. Carcinoid tumors. N Engl J Med 1999;340(11):858–68.
31. Lundin L, Norheim I, Landelius J, et al. Carcinoid heart disease: relationship of circulating vasoactive substances to ultrasound-detectable cardiac abnormalities. Circulation 1988;77(2):264–9.
32. Robiolio PA, Rigolin VH, Wilson JS, et al. Carcinoid heart disease. Correlation of high serotonin levels with valvular abnormalities detected by cardiac catheterization and echocardiography. Circulation 1995;92(4):790–5.
33. Yoon SN, Yu CS, Shin US, et al. Clinicopathological characteristics of rectal carcinoids. Int J Colorectal Dis 2010;25(9):1087–92.
34. Weinstock B, Ward SC, Harpaz N, et al. Clinical and prognostic features of rectal neuroendocrine tumors. Neuroendocrinology 2013;98(3):180–7.
35. Lawrence B, Gustafsson BI, Chan A, et al. The epidemiology of gastroenteropancreatic neuroendocrine tumors. Endocrinol Metab Clin North Am 2011; 40(1):1–18, vii.
36. Lawrence B, Kidd M, Svejda B, et al. A clinical perspective on gastric neuroendocrine neoplasia. Curr Gastroenterol Rep 2011;13(1):101–9.

37. Basuroy R, Srirajaskanthan R, Prachalias A, et al. Review article: the investigation and management of gastric neuroendocrine tumours. Aliment Pharmacol Ther 2014;39(10):1071–84.

38. Modlin IM, Moss SF, Gustafsson BI, et al. The archaic distinction between functioning and nonfunctioning neuroendocrine neoplasms is no longer clinically relevant. Langenbecks Arch Surg 2011;396(8):1145–56.

39. Kulke MH, Bendell J, Kvols L, et al. Evolving diagnostic and treatment strategies for pancreatic neuroendocrine tumors. J Hematol Oncol 2011;4:29.

40. Tan EH, Tan CH. Imaging of gastroenteropancreatic neuroendocrine tumors. World J Clin Oncol 2011;2(1):28–43.

41. Noone TC, Hosey J, Firat Z, et al. Imaging and localization of islet-cell tumours of the pancreas on CT and MRI. Best Pract Res Clin Endocrinol Metab 2005;19(2):195–211.

42. Paulson EK, Mcdermott VG, Keogan MT, et al. Carcinoid metastases to the liver: role of triple-phase helical CT. Radiology 1998;206(1):143–50.

43. Owen NJ, Sohaib SA, Peppercorn PD, et al. MRI of pancreatic neuroendocrine tumours. Br J Radiol 2001;74(886):968–73.

44. Semelka RC, Custodio CM, Cem Balci N, et al. Neuroendocrine tumors of the pancreas: spectrum of appearances on MRI. J Magn Reson Imaging 2000;11(2):141–8.

45. Bader TR, Semelka RC, Chiu VC, et al. MRI of carcinoid tumors: spectrum of appearances in the gastrointestinal tract and liver. J Magn Reson Imaging 2001;14(3):261–9.

46. Dromain C, De Baere T, Baudin E, et al. MR imaging of hepatic metastases caused by neuroendocrine tumors: comparing four techniques. AJR Am J Roentgenol 2003;180(1):121–8.

47. Liapi E, Geschwind JF, Vossen JA, et al. Functional MRI evaluation of tumor response in patients with neuroendocrine hepatic metastasis treated with transcatheter arterial chemoembolization. AJR Am J Roentgenol 2008;190(1):67–73.

48. Anaye A, Mathieu A, Closset J, et al. Successful preoperative localization of a small pancreatic insulinoma by diffusion-weighted MRI. JOP 2009;10(5):528–31.

49. Lee SS, Byun JH, Park BJ, et al. Quantitative analysis of diffusion-weighted magnetic resonance imaging of the pancreas: usefulness in characterizing solid pancreatic masses. J Magn Reson Imaging 2008;28(4):928–36.

50. Fjallskog ML, Ludvigsen E, Stridsberg M, et al. Expression of somatostatin receptor subtypes 1 to 5 in tumor tissue and intratumoral vessels in malignant endocrine pancreatic tumors. Med Oncol 2003;20(1):59–67.

51. Kaemmerer D, Peter L, Lupp A, et al. Comparing of IRS and Her2 as immunohistochemical scoring schemes in gastroenteropancreatic neuroendocrine tumors. Int J Clin Exp Pathol 2012;5(3):187–94.

52. Teunissen JJ, Kwekkeboom DJ, Valkema R, et al. Nuclear medicine techniques for the imaging and treatment of neuroendocrine tumours. Endocr Relat Cancer 2011;18(Suppl 1):S27–51.

53. Geijer H, Breimer LH. Somatostatin receptor PET/CT in neuroendocrine tumours: update on systematic review and meta-analysis. Eur J Nucl Med Mol Imaging 2013;40(11):1770–80.

54. Binderup T, Knigge U, Loft A, et al. Functional imaging of neuroendocrine tumors: a head-to-head comparison of somatostatin receptor scintigraphy, 123I-MIBG scintigraphy, and 18F-FDG PET. J Nucl Med 2010;51(5):704–12.

55. Basuroy R, Sarker D, Quaglia A, et al. Personalized medicine for gastroentero-pancreatic neuroendocrine tumors: a distant dream? Int J Endocr Oncol 2015; 2(3):201–15.

56. Khan MS, Kirkwood A, Tsigani T, et al. Circulating tumor cells as prognostic markers in neuroendocrine tumors. J Clin Oncol 2013;31(3):365–72.

57. Modlin IM, Frilling A, Salem RR, et al. Blood measurement of neuroendocrine gene transcripts defines the effectiveness of operative resection and ablation strategies. Surgery 2016;159(1):336–47.

58. Bodei L, Kidd M, Modlin IM, et al. Measurement of circulating transcripts and gene cluster analysis predicts and defines therapeutic efficacy of peptide receptor radionuclide therapy (PRRT) in neuroendocrine tumors. Eur J Nucl Med Mol Imaging 2015;43(5):839–51.

59. Cwikla JB, Bodei L, Kolasinska-Cwikla A, et al. Circulating transcript analysis (NETest) in GEP-NETs treated with somatostatin analogs defines therapy. J Clin Endocrinol Metab 2015;100(11):E1437–45.

60. Lawrence B, Gustafsson BI, Kidd M, et al. The clinical relevance of chromogranin A as a biomarker for gastroenteropancreatic neuroendocrine tumors. Endocrinol Metab Clin North Am 2011;40(1):111–34, viii.

61. Arnold R, Wilke A, Rinke A, et al. Plasma chromogranin A as marker for survival in patients with metastatic endocrine gastroenteropancreatic tumors. Clin Gastroenterol Hepatol 2008;6(7):820–7.

62. Durante C, Boukheris H, Dromain C, et al. Prognostic factors influencing survival from metastatic (stage IV) gastroenteropancreatic well-differentiated endocrine carcinoma. Endocr Relat Cancer 2009;16(2):585–97.

63. Yang X, Yang Y, Li Z, et al. Diagnostic value of circulating chromogranin a for neuroendocrine tumors: a systematic review and meta-analysis. PLoS One 2015;10(4):e0124884.

64. Modlin IM, Shapiro MD, Kidd M. Siegfried Oberndorfer: origins and perspectives of carcinoid tumors. Hum Pathol 2004;35(12):1440–51.

65. Crippa S, Partelli S, Bassi C, et al. Long-term outcomes and prognostic factors in neuroendocrine carcinomas of the pancreas: morphology matters. Surgery 2016;159(3):862–71.

66. Capurso G, Bettini R, Rinzivillo M, et al. Role of resection of the primary pancreatic neuroendocrine tumour only in patients with unresectable metastatic liver disease: a systematic review. Neuroendocrinology 2011;93(4):223–9.

67. Srirajaskanthan R, Ahmed A, Prachialias A, et al. ENETS TNM staging predicts prognosis in small bowel neuroendocrine tumours. ISRN Oncol 2013;2013: 420795.

68. Ahmed A, Turner G, King B, et al. Midgut neuroendocrine tumours with liver metastases: results of the UKINETS study. Endocr Relat Cancer 2009;16(3): 885–94.

69. Farley HA, Pommier RF. Surgical treatment of small bowel neuroendocrine tumors. Hematol Oncol Clin North Am 2016;30(1):49–61.

70. Frilling A, Li J, Malamutmann E, et al. Treatment of liver metastases from neuroendocrine tumours in relation to the extent of hepatic disease. Br J Surg 2009; 96(2):175–84.

71. Basuroy R, Srirajaskanthan R, Ramage JK. A multimodal approach to the management of neuroendocrine tumour liver metastases. Int J Hepatol 2012;2012: 819193.

72. Chamberlain RS, Canes D, Brown KT, et al. Hepatic neuroendocrine metastases: does intervention alter outcomes? J Am Coll Surg 2000;190(4):432–45.

73. Que FG, Nagorney DM, Batts KP, et al. Hepatic resection for metastatic neuro-endocrine carcinomas. Am J Surg 1995;169(1):36–42 [discussion: 42–3].

74. Gurusamy KS, Ramamoorthy R, Sharma D, et al. Liver resection versus other treatments for neuroendocrine tumours in patients with resectable liver metasta-ses. Cochrane Database Syst Rev 2009;(2):CD007060.

75. Gurusamy KS, Pamecha V, Sharma D, et al. Palliative cytoreductive surgery versus other palliative treatments in patients with unresectable liver metastases from gastro-entero-pancreatic neuroendocrine tumours. Cochrane Database Syst Rev 2009;(1):CD007118.

76. Frilling A, Modlin IM, Kidd M, et al. Recommendations for management of pa-tients with neuroendocrine liver metastases. Lancet Oncol 2014;15(1):e8–21.

77. Gillams A, Cassoni A, Conway G, et al. Radiofrequency ablation of neuroendo-crine liver metastases: the Middlesex experience. Abdom Imaging 2005;30(4): 435–41.

78. Gupta S, Johnson MM, Murthy R, et al. Hepatic arterial embolization and chemoembolization for the treatment of patients with metastatic neuroendocrine tumors: variables affecting response rates and survival. Cancer 2005;104(8): 1590–602.

79. Toumpanakis C, Meyer T, Caplin ME. Cytotoxic treatment including emboliza-tion/chemoembolization for neuroendocrine tumours. Best Pract Res Clin Endo-crinol Metab 2007;21(1):131–44.

80. Ruszniewski P, Rougier P, Roche A, et al. Hepatic arterial chemoembolization in patients with liver metastases of endocrine tumors. A prospective phase II study in 24 patients. Cancer 1993;71(8):2624–30.

81. Therasse E, Breittmayer F, Roche A, et al. Transcatheter chemoembolization of progressive carcinoid liver metastasis. Radiology 1993;189(2):541–7.

82. Clouse ME, Perry L, Stuart K, et al. Hepatic arterial chemoembolization for met-astatic neuroendocrine tumors. Digestion 1994;55(Suppl 3):92–7.

83. Diaco DS, Hajarizadeh H, Mueller CR, et al. Treatment of metastatic carcinoid tumors using multimodality therapy of octreotide acetate, intra-arterial chemo-therapy, and hepatic arterial chemoembolization. Am J Surg 1995;169(5):523–8.

84. Roche A, Girish BV, De Baere T, et al. Trans-catheter arterial chemoembolization as first-line treatment for hepatic metastases from endocrine tumors. Eur Radiol 2003;13(1):136–40.

85. Kim YH, Ajani JA, Carrasco CH, et al. Selective hepatic arterial chemoemboliza-tion for liver metastases in patients with carcinoid tumor or islet cell carcinoma. Cancer Invest 1999;17(7):474–8.

86. Drougas JG, Anthony LB, Blair TK, et al. Hepatic artery chemoembolization for management of patients with advanced metastatic carcinoid tumors. Am J Surg 1998;175(5):408–12.

87. Marrache F, Vullierme MP, Roy C, et al. Arterial phase enhancement and body mass index are predictors of response to chemoembolisation for liver metasta-ses of endocrine tumours. Br J Cancer 2007;96(1):49–55.

88. Stubbs RS, Cannan RJ, Mitchell AW. Selective internal radiation therapy (SIRT) with 90Yttrium microspheres for extensive colorectal liver metastases. Hepato-gastroenterology 2001;48(38):333–7.

89. Kennedy AS, Dezarn WA, Mcneillie P, et al. Radioembolization for unresectable neuroendocrine hepatic metastases using resin 90Y-microspheres: early results in 148 patients. Am J Clin Oncol 2008;31(3):271–9.

90. King J, Quinn R, Glenn DM, et al. Radioembolization with selective internal radiation microspheres for neuroendocrine liver metastases. Cancer 2008;113(5): 921–9.

91. Murthy R, Kamat P, Nunez R, et al. Yttrium-90 microsphere radioembolotherapy of hepatic metastatic neuroendocrine carcinomas after hepatic arterial embolization. J Vasc Interv Radiol 2008;19(1):145–51.

92. Barbier CE, Garske-Roman U, Sandstrom M, et al. Selective internal radiation therapy in patients with progressive neuroendocrine liver metastases. Eur J Nucl Med Mol Imaging 2015;1–7.

93. Lamberts SW, Van Der Lely AJ, De Herder WW, et al. Octreotide. N Engl J Med 1996;334(4):246–54.

94. Shah T, Caplin M. Endocrine tumours of the gastrointestinal tract. Biotherapy for metastatic endocrine tumours. Best Pract Res Clin Gastroenterol 2005;19(4): 617–36.

95. O'toole D, Ducreux M, Bommelaer G, et al. Treatment of carcinoid syndrome: a prospective crossover evaluation of lanreotide versus octreotide in terms of efficacy, patient acceptability, and tolerance. Cancer 2000;88(4):770–6.

96. Oberg K, Kvols L, Caplin M, et al. Consensus report on the use of somatostatin analogs for the management of neuroendocrine tumors of the gastroenteropancreatic system. Ann Oncol 2004;15(6):966–73.

97. Plockinger U, Wiedenmann B. Neuroendocrine tumors. Biotherapy. Best Pract Res Clin Endocrinol Metab 2007;21(1):145–62.

98. Rinke A, Muller HH, Schade-Brittinger C, et al. Placebo-controlled, double-blind, prospective, randomized study on the effect of octreotide LAR in the control of tumor growth in patients with metastatic neuroendocrine midgut tumors: a report from the PROMID Study Group. J Clin Oncol 2009;27(28):4656–63.

99. Caplin ME, Pavel M, Cwikla JB, et al. Lanreotide in metastatic enteropancreatic neuroendocrine tumors. N Engl J Med 2014;371(3):224–33.

100. Wolin EM, Jarzab B, Eriksson B, et al. Phase III study of pasireotide long-acting release in patients with metastatic neuroendocrine tumors and carcinoid symptoms refractory to available somatostatin analogues. Drug Des Devel Ther 2015; 9:5075–86.

101. Moertel CG, Hanley JA, Johnson LA. Streptozocin alone compared with streptozocin plus fluorouracil in the treatment of advanced islet-cell carcinoma. N Engl J Med 1980;303(21):1189–94.

102. Meyer T, Qian W, Caplin ME, et al. Capecitabine and streptozocin ± cisplatin in advanced gastroenteropancreatic neuroendocrine tumours. Eur J Cancer 2014; 50(5):902–11.

103. Ekeblad S, Sundin A, Janson ET, et al. Temozolomide as monotherapy is effective in treatment of advanced malignant neuroendocrine tumors. Clin Cancer Res 2007;13(10):2986–91.

104. Strosberg J. Advances in the treatment of pancreatic neuroendocrine tumors (pNETs). Gastrointest Cancer Res 2013;6(4 Suppl 1):S10–2.

105. Kulke MH, Kim H, Clark JW, et al. A phase II trial of gemcitabine for metastatic neuroendocrine tumors. Cancer 2004;101(5):934–9.

106. Moertel CG, Lefkopoulo M, Lipsitz S, et al. Streptozocin-doxorubicin, streptozocin-fluorouracil or chlorozotocin in the treatment of advanced islet-cell carcinoma. N Engl J Med 1992;326(8):519–23.

107. Eriksson B, Skogseid B, Lundqvist G, et al. Medical treatment and long-term survival in a prospective study of 84 patients with endocrine pancreatic tumors. Cancer 1990;65(9):1883–90.

108. Moertel CG, Hanley JA. Combination chemotherapy trials in metastatic carcinoid tumor and the malignant carcinoid syndrome. Cancer Clin Trials 1979; 2(4):327–34.

109. Sun W, Lipsitz S, Catalano P, et al, Eastern Cooperative Oncology Group. Phase II/III study of doxorubicin with fluorouracil compared with streptozocin with fluorouracil or dacarbazine in the treatment of advanced carcinoid tumors: Eastern Cooperative Oncology Group Study E1281. J Clin Oncol 2005;23(22):4897–904.

110. Kulke MH, Wu B, Ryan DP, et al. A phase II trial of irinotecan and cisplatin in patients with metastatic neuroendocrine tumors. Dig Dis Sci 2006;51(6):1033–8.

111. Rivera E, Ajani JA. Doxorubicin, streptozocin, and 5-fluorouracil chemotherapy for patients with metastatic islet-cell carcinoma. Am J Clin Oncol 1998;21(1): 36–8.

112. Kulke MH, Stuart K, Enzinger PC, et al. Phase II study of temozolomide and thalidomide in patients with metastatic neuroendocrine tumors. J Clin Oncol 2006;24(3):401–6.

113. Moertel CG, Kvols LK, O'connell MJ, et al. Treatment of neuroendocrine carcinomas with combined etoposide and cisplatin. Evidence of major therapeutic activity in the anaplastic variants of these neoplasms. Cancer 1991;68(2): 227–32.

114. Mitry E, Baudin E, Ducreux M, et al. Treatment of poorly differentiated neuroendocrine tumours with etoposide and cisplatin. Br J Cancer 1999;81(8):1351–5.

115. Mani MA, Shroff RT, Jacobs C, et al. A phase II study of irinotecan and cisplatin for metastatic or unresectable high grade neuroendocrine carcinoma. J Clin Oncol 2008;26(15S):15550.

116. Kwekkeboom DJ, De Herder WW, Kam BL, et al. Treatment with the radiolabeled somatostatin analog [177 Lu-DOTA 0,Tyr3]octreotate: toxicity, efficacy, and survival. J Clin Oncol 2008;26(13):2124–30.

117. Strosberg JR, Wolin EM, Chasen B, et al. NETTER-1 phase III: Progression-free survival, radiographic response, and preliminary overall survival results in patients with midgut neuroendocrine tumors treated with 177-Lu-Dotatate. J Clin Oncol 34, 2016 (suppl 4S; abstr 194).

118. Kwekkeboom DJ, Teunissen JJ, Bakker WH, et al. Radiolabeled somatostatin analog [177Lu-DOTA0,Tyr3]octreotate in patients with endocrine gastroenteropancreatic tumors. J Clin Oncol 2005;23(12):2754–62.

119. Van Essen M, Krenning EP, De Jong M, et al. Peptide receptor radionuclide therapy with radiolabelled somatostatin analogues in patients with somatostatin receptor positive tumours. Acta Oncol 2007;46(6):723–34.

120. Bodei L, Cremonesi M, Ferrari M, et al. Long-term evaluation of renal toxicity after peptide receptor radionuclide therapy with 90Y-DOTATOC and 177Lu-DOTATATE: the role of associated risk factors. Eur J Nucl Med Mol Imaging 2008; 35(10):1847–56.

121. Hoefnagel CA, De Kraker J, Valdes Olmos RA, et al. 131I-MIBG as a first-line treatment in high-risk neuroblastoma patients. Nucl Med Commun 1994;15(9): 712–7.

122. Taal BG, Hoefnagel CA, Valdes Olmos RA, et al. Palliative effect of metaiodobenzylguanidine in metastatic carcinoid tumors. J Clin Oncol 1996;14(6): 1829–38.

123. Pathirana AA, Vinjamuri S, Byrne C, et al. (131)I-MIBG radionuclide therapy is safe and cost-effective in the control of symptoms of the carcinoid syndrome. Eur J Surg Oncol 2001;27(4):404–8.

124. Mukherjee JJ, Kaltsas GA, Islam N, et al. Treatment of metastatic carcinoid tumours, phaeochromocytoma, paraganglioma and medullary carcinoma of the thyroid with (131)I-meta-iodobenzylguanidine [(131)I-mIBG]. Clin Endocrinol (Oxf) 2001;55(1):47–60.

125. Bomanji J, Britton KE, Ur E, et al. Treatment of malignant phaeochromocytoma, paraganglioma and carcinoid tumours with 131I-metaiodobenzylguanidine. Nucl Med Commun 1993;14(10):856–61.

126. Buscombe JR, Cwikla JB, Caplin ME, et al. Long-term efficacy of low activity meta-[131I]iodobenzylguanidine therapy in patients with disseminated neuroendocrine tumours depends on initial response. Nucl Med Commun 2005;26(11): 969–76.

127. Mulholland N, Chakravartty R, Devlin L, et al. Long-term outcomes of (131) Iodine mIBG therapy in metastatic gastrointestinal pancreatic neuroendocrine tumours: single administration predicts non-responders. Eur J Nucl Med Mol Imaging 2015;42(13):2002–12.

128. Otte A, Herrmann R, Heppeler A, et al. Yttrium-90 DOTATOC: first clinical results. Eur J Nucl Med 1999;26(11):1439–47.

129. Waldherr C, Pless M, Maecke HR, et al. Tumor response and clinical benefit in neuroendocrine tumors after 7.4 GBq (90)Y-DOTATOC. J Nucl Med 2002;43(5): 610–6.

130. Valkema R, Pauwels S, Kvols LK, et al. Survival and response after peptide receptor radionuclide therapy with [90Y-DOTA0,Tyr3]octreotide in patients with advanced gastroenteropancreatic neuroendocrine tumors. Semin Nucl Med 2006;36(2):147–56.

131. Yang Q, Guan KL. Expanding mTOR signaling. Cell Res 2007;17(8):666–81.

132. Capdevila J, Salazar R, Halperin I, et al. Innovations therapy: mammalian target of rapamycin (mTOR) inhibitors for the treatment of neuroendocrine tumors. Cancer Metastasis Rev 2011;30(Suppl 1):27–34.

133. Yao JC, Fazio N, Singh S, et al. Everolimus for the treatment of advanced, non-functional neuroendocrine tumours of the lung or gastrointestinal tract (RADIANT-4): a randomised, placebo-controlled, phase 3 study. Lancet 2015; 387(10022):968–77.

134. Raymond E, Dahan L, Raoul JL, et al. Sunitinib malate for the treatment of pancreatic neuroendocrine tumors. N Engl J Med 2011;364(6):501–13.

# Heritable Gastrointestinal Cancer Syndromes

Elena M. Stoffel, MD, MPH

## KEYWORDS

- Gastrointestinal cancer • Genetics • Hereditary syndromes

## KEY POINTS

- Although almost all gastrointestinal cancers develop as a consequence of sporadic genomic events, approximately 5% arise in the setting of germline mutations in genes known to be associated with cancer predisposition.
- The number of genes associated with heritable cancer syndromes continues to increase, and tumor phenotypes, along with family history, provide the framework for identifying individuals at risk.
- Making the diagnosis of a hereditary cancer syndrome has implications for management of patients with gastrointestinal neoplasia and for their family members.
- Systematic approaches that integrate family history and molecular characterization of tumors and polyps can facilitate identification of individuals with genetic predisposition to gastrointestinal cancer.

## GENES AND CANCER

Like most other cancers, gastrointestinal neoplasms arise as a consequence of the deregulation of signaling pathways controlling cell survival and genome maintenance.[1] In almost all tumors, genetic mutations that affect the function of genes involved in key cell regulatory functions (eg, tumor suppression and DNA repair) occur sporadically in individual cells as so-called somatic events. However, a small proportion of individuals harbor mutations in their germline DNA that predispose to the development of gastrointestinal neoplasms. Because epithelial cells of the digestive tract are among the most rapidly dividing cells in the human body, germline mutations in a variety of cancer genes can be associated with dramatic increases in risk for gastrointestinal tumors.

Identification of the various heritable syndromes associated with risk for gastrointestinal neoplasia has come about through meticulous study of hundreds of individuals belonging to cancer families. Categorization of clinical histories and tumor phenotypes has led to the identification of specific hereditary cancer syndromes and the germline

Disclosures: None.
Division of Gastroenterology, Department of Internal Medicine, University of Michigan Health System, 2150A Cancer Center, Ann Arbor, MI 48109, USA
*E-mail address:* estoffel@med.umich.edu

**Table 1**
Heritable cancer syndromes associated with predisposition to gastrointestinal cancers

| Syndrome | Genes | Estimated Carrier Frequency (General Population) | CRC | Gastric | Small Bowel | Pancreatic | Breast | Ovarian | Endometrial |
|---|---|---|---|---|---|---|---|---|---|
| | | | | | | Lifetime Cancer Risks | | | |
| Lynch Syndrome | MLH1, MSH2, MSH6, PMS2, EPCAM | 1 in 280–350 | e | b | — | a | a | b | d |
| Familial Adenomatous Polyposis | APC | 1 in 1000 | e | a | b | — | — | — | — |
| MUTYH-Associated Polyposis | MUTYH | 1 in 100 | c | — | — | — | — | — | — |
| Li Fraumeni Syndrome | P53 | — | b | b | | a | c | — | — |
| Juvenile Polyposis | SMAD4 BMPR1A | — | c | b | | a | — | — | — |
| Peutz-Jeghers Syndrome | STK11 | — | c | b | a | c | d | — | — |
| Cowden or PTEN Hamartoma Tumor Syndrome | PTEN | — | b | — | — | — | c | — | c |
| Hereditary Diffuse Gastric Cancer | CDH1 | — | a,b | e | — | — | d | — | — |
| Hereditary Breast Ovarian Cancer Syndrome | BRCA1 BRCA2 PALB2 | — | — | — | — | a / TBD | e / c | c / a | — |
| Familial Atypical Multiple Mole Melanoma | CDKN2A | — | — | — | — | b | — | — | — |

*Abbreviation:* TBD, to be determined.
[a] 2% to 5%.
[b] 5% to 20%.
[c] 21% to 40%.
[d] 41% to 60%.
[e] Greater than 60%.

*Adapted from* Stoffel EM. Screening in GI cancers: the role of genetics. J Clin Oncol 2015;33(16):1722; with permission.

DNA alterations corresponding to each (**Table 1**). Personal and family history remains the primary components of clinical algorithms used for cancer risk stratification. However, variability in penetrance and expressivity associated with heritable gene mutations can make family history imprecise and approaches that integrate tumor histopathology and molecular phenotype with family history offer the opportunity to most effectively identify individuals with genetic predisposition to cancer. Because advances in genomic technologies promise to make tumor profiling routine as a strategy for selecting treatments, this information can also be used to identify individuals whose cancers arise as a consequence of germline mutations associated with cancer predisposition. The implementation of universal screening of colorectal cancer (CRC) for DNA mismatch repair (MMR) deficiency is effective not only in guiding oncologic therapies but also in identifying CRC patients affected with Lynch syndrome.[2] Furthermore, there are additional histopathologic subtypes of gastrointestinal cancers (eg, signet ring cell gastric cancers, pancreatic cancers with somatic *BRCA1* or *BRCA2* mutations) for which genetic evaluation should be considered.

This article presents an overview of heritable cancer syndromes associated with risk for gastrointestinal cancers, and outlines strategies for diagnosis and management of at-risk individuals.

## COLORECTAL CANCER

CRC is the third most common cancer affecting men and women in the United States, with the average individual having a lifetime risk of 5%. Family history is among the strongest predictors of risk for CRC; consequently, current algorithms for CRC screening and surveillance rely heavily on family history of CRC to determine age to begin screening and surveillance intervals.[3] Approximately 1 in 3 individuals diagnosed with CRC reports a diagnosis of CRC in a close relative and, on average, 1 in 20 CRC patients carries a germline mutation associated with a heritable cancer syndrome.[4] The National Comprehensive Cancer Network (NCCN) criteria for identifying individuals for whom genetic referral should be considered for evaluation for genetic syndromes associated with CRC risk are presented in **Box 1**.[5] Although routine implementation of CRC screening among individuals age 50 years and older has resulted in overall reductions of CRC-related incidence and mortality, incidence of CRC among individuals age less than 50 years continues to rise by 1.5% per year.[6] The prevalence

---

**Box 1**
**National Comprehensive Cancer Network criteria for further risk evaluation for high-risk syndromes associated with colorectal cancer**

1. Individuals meeting the revised Bethesda guidelines

2. Individuals meeting the Amsterdam criteria

3. Individuals with greater than 20 colorectal adenomas

4. Individuals with multiple gastrointestinal hamartomatous polyps or serrated polyposis

5. Individuals from a family with a known hereditary syndrome associated with CRC with or without a known mutation

6. Individuals with desmoid tumor, cribriform-morular variant of papillary thyroid cancer, or hepatoblastoma

*Data from* National Comprehensive Cancer Network. Genetic/Familial high-risk assessment: colorectal. NCCN clinical practice guidelines in oncology 2015. v. 2.2015. Available at: nccn. org. Accessed April 13, 2016.

of germline mutations associated with cancer predisposition is higher among individuals diagnosed at young ages and studies suggest many of these do not meet the classic diagnostic criteria for the associated syndrome.[7] Several hereditary cancer syndromes confer lifetime risks of CRC that exceed 50% in the absence of medical or surgical intervention, justifying the importance of presymptomatic diagnosis for these high-risk individuals.

Family history has long been a cornerstone for CRC risk assessment and identification of individuals at risk for hereditary CRC. The Amsterdam criteria ($\geq$3 relatives diagnosed with CRC, in 2 or more consecutive generations, with at least 1 case diagnosed at age <50 years) were originally developed for research purposes to identify individuals with presumed autosomal dominant inherited predisposition syndromes.[8] Although the Amsterdam criteria have proven invaluable in identifying families with germline mutations in DNA MMR genes associated with Lynch syndrome, observations that fewer than half of families with genetically confirmed Lynch syndrome meet the Amsterdam criteria[9] and that 1 in 4 individuals with germline MMR mutations have atypical family histories[10] illustrate the limited sensitivity of family history of cancer for identifying individuals with heritable cancer syndromes.

Tumor analysis offers another avenue for identifying individuals with genetic predisposition to cancer. CRCs develop through different molecular pathways (eg, chromosomal instability, DNA MMR deficiency, and aberrant DNA methylation) that are associated with differences in treatment responses and prognosis; consequently molecular profiling of CRCs for somatic mutations in *BRAF*, *KRAS*, and DNA MMR status has been integrated into standard algorithms used to guide therapy.[11] Universal screening of CRC tumors for DNA MMR deficiency associated with Lynch syndrome is the starting point for clinical algorithms used to stratify CRC patients with regard to risk for heritable cancer syndromes (**Fig. 1**).

### Lynch Syndrome

Lynch syndrome, also known as hereditary nonpolyposis CRC (HNPCC), is responsible for 3% of all CRC cases, making it the most common heritable syndrome associated with risk for CRC.[10] The molecular basis of Lynch syndrome is germline mutations in 1 of the DNA MMR genes (*MLH1*, *MSH2*, *MSH6*, *PMS2*, or *EPCAM*) that lead to accumulation of mutations and development of tumors, which exhibit high levels of DNA microsatellite instability (MSI)-H. The carrier rate of germline MMR mutations is estimated to be 1 in 280 to 440 in the general population.[12] CRC is the most common cancer affecting MMR mutation carriers, with lifetime risk of CRC ranging from 22% to 75% and endometrial cancer risks for women ranging from 32% to 45%.[13–17] Risks for additional extracolonic cancers are also increased for carriers of DNA MMR germline mutations, among these ovarian, gastric, small intestinal, urinary tract, brain, pancreatic, and sebaceous neoplasms of the skin.

### Diagnosis

Identification of individuals at risk for Lynch syndrome involves assessment of personal and family history and tumor phenotypes, and the diagnosis is confirmed once a pathogenic mutation in a DNA MMR gene (*MLH1*, *MSH2*, *MSH6*, *PMS2*, or *EPCAM*) is identified through testing of germline DNA. Clinical guidelines (eg, Amsterdam criteria, Bethesda guidelines[18]) and risk prediction models (eg, MMRPro,[12] PREMM1,2,6[19]) have been used for identifying carriers of MMR mutations based on personal and family history; however, universal screening of all CRC tumors for MMR deficiency has been shown to be the most sensitive and cost-effective strategy for identifying individuals with Lynch syndrome.[2,20]

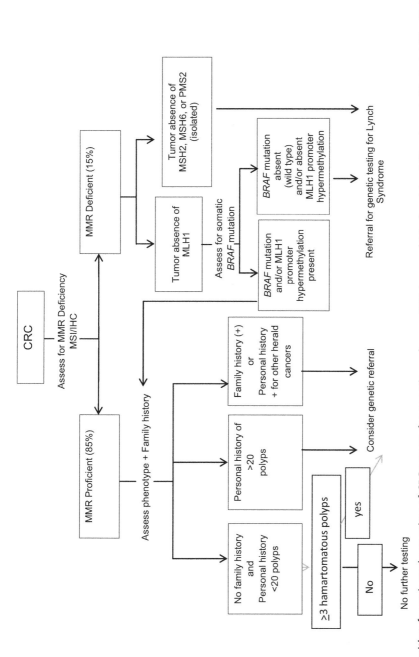

**Fig. 1.** Algorithm for universal screening of CRC tumors for genetic syndromes. IHC, immunohistochemistry; MSI, microsatellite instability. (*Adapted from* Stoffel EM, Boland CR. Genetics and genetic testing in hereditary colorectal cancer. Gastroenterology 2015;149(5):1198; with permission.)

**Tumor screening** CRC tumors can be screened for MMR deficiency using polymerase chain reaction–based testing for instability at DNA MSI or through immunohistochemistry (IHC) staining for DNA MMR proteins MLH1, MSH2, MSH6, and PMS2. Absence of expression of 1 or more MMR proteins is considered diagnostic of MMR deficiency. Approximately 15% of CRCs are MMR-deficient, with most of these exhibiting loss of MLH1 or PMS2 protein expression as a result of somatic mutations in BRAF or MLH1 promoter hypermethylation. Individuals whose tumors exhibit either loss of MSH2 and/or MSH6 proteins, or loss of MLH1 and/or PMS2 in the absence of somatic *BRAF* mutations or MLH1 promoter hypermethylation should be tested for germline mutations in MMR genes to confirm the diagnosis of Lynch syndrome. Lynch syndrome can be implicated in approximately 3% of all CRCs, and most Lynch syndrome–associated CRCs are MMR-deficient. Although sensitivity of either MSI or IHC individually for identifying individuals with Lynch syndrome ranges from 77% to 90%, results can be discordant, and false negatives can occur, especially in CRCs associated with germline mutations in *MSH6*.[21] Although tumor screening of endometrial cancers has similar performance characteristics to CRC, testing of other neoplasms (eg, ovarian cancers, colorectal adenomas[22]) for MMR deficiency may be less sensitive.

## Management

Making a diagnosis of Lynch syndrome has significant implications for clinical management for patients who have cancer and their at-risk relatives. Lynch syndrome–associated colorectal neoplasms develop at young ages and exhibit accelerated adenoma-carcinoma progression compared with sporadic CRC, thus specialized surveillance is required with colonoscopy every 1 to 2 years beginning at age 20 to 25 years.[20,23] Given the high risk for endometrial cancer, it is recommended that women begin annual surveillance with endometrial biopsy and transvaginal ultrasound starting at age 30 to 35 years, with consideration for prophylactic hysterectomy once childbearing has been completed (**Box 2**).[20,23]

For individuals diagnosed with CRC, the high risk for metachronous CRC justifies consideration of a more extensive surgical resection (eg, subtotal colectomy).[20] Furthermore, observations that Lynch syndrome–associated CRCs may have a less favorable response to treatment with 5-fluorouracil[24] and that advanced MSI-H CRCs may respond well to programmed cell death-1 inhibitors[25] has implications for oncologic therapies.

Once the diagnosis of Lynch syndrome has been made, patients should be instructed to share this information with at-risk family members who may benefit from predisposition genetic testing and/or enhanced surveillance. Population-based screening for Lynch syndrome can be cost-effective and models estimate that between 3 to 4 asymptomatic relatives need to be tested for each germline mutation carrier identified.[26]

## COLONIC POLYPOSIS SYNDROMES
### Familial Adenomatous Polyposis

Although familial adenomatous polyposis (FAP) accounts for only 1% of all CRCs,[4] it is perhaps the most readily recognizable of the heritable syndromes based on its classic phenotype of 100s to 1000s of colorectal polyps. For individuals with the classic phenotype, the lifetime risk for CRC may exceed 90% in the absence of proctocolectomy. Although the colorectal polyposis is the most distinctive manifestation, adenomas can develop in the duodenum and ampulla. Risk for thyroid cancer is

| Box 2 | |
|---|---|
| **Recommended cancer surveillance for individuals at risk for heritable gastrointestinal cancers** | |
| **Syndrome** | **Management** |
| Lynch syndrome | Colonoscopy every 1–2 years starting at age 20–25 years |
| | Consider upper endoscopy every 3–5 years |
| | Consider endometrial cancer screening (transvaginal ultrasound and/or endometrial biopsy) starting at age 30–35 years or prophylactic hysterectomy after completion of childbearing (women) |
| Familial adenomatous polyposis | |
|    Classic | Colonoscopy every 1–2 years, starting at age 10–12 years, colectomy for large polyp burden |
| | Upper endoscopy every 6 months to 4 years |
| | Consider annual thyroid ultrasound |
|    Attenuated | Colonoscopy every 1–2 years, beginning in late adolescence |
| | Consider upper endoscopy |
| *MUTYH*-associated polyposis | Colonoscopy every 1–2 years, starting at age 20–25 years |
| | Upper endoscopy every 1–3 years |
| | Consider thyroid ultrasound |
| Peutz-Jeghers syndrome | Upper endoscopy every 2–3 years starting at age 8–10 years |
| | Small bowel (capsule endoscopy or CT/MR enterography) every 1–3 years starting at age 8–10 years |
| | Colonoscopy every 2–3 years, starting in teenage years |
| | Pancreas screening (MR cholangiopancreatography or EUS) every 1–2 years, starting at age 35 years. |
| | Mammogram and breast MRI, yearly, starting at age 25 years |
| | Testicular examination or ultrasound yearly (men) |
| | Transvaginal ultrasound, yearly, starting at age 18–25 years (women) |
| Juvenile polyposis | Upper endoscopy every 1–3 years starting age 15 years |
| | Colonoscopy every 1–3 years starting age 15 years |
| | SMAD4 mutation carriers should have screening for hereditary hemorrhagic telangiectasia |
| Cowden syndrome | Colonoscopy every 3–5 years, beginning age 30–35 years |
| | Upper endoscopy, interval depends on polyp burden |
| | Mammogram and breast MRI, yearly, starting at age 25 years |
| | Endometrial cancer screening with transvaginal ultrasound and/or endometrial biopsy starting age 30–35 years (women) |
| | Thyroid ultrasound (annual) |
| | Consider renal ultrasound (annually) |
| Familial colorectal cancer type X | Colonoscopy every 3–5 years |
| | Beginning age 30–35 years |
| Serrated polyposis | Colonoscopy every 1–3 years depending on polyp burden |
| Hereditary diffuse gastric cancer | Upper endoscopy annually beginning in late adolescence |
| | Consider prophylactic total gastrectomy after age 20 years |
| | Consider colonoscopy |
| | Breast screening with mammogram and breast MRI annually starting at age 25 years |
| Genetic predisposition to pancreatic cancer | Endoscopic ultrasound alternating with MR cholangiopancreatography (annual), beginning at age 50 years or 10 years earlier than relatives' diagnosis |

*Adapted from* Syngal S, Brand RE, Church JM, et al. ACG clinical guideline: genetic testing and management of hereditary gastrointestinal cancer sydromes. Am J Gastroenterol 2015;110(2):223–62; and Giardiello FM, Allen JI, Axilbund JE, et al. Guidelines on genetic evaluation and management of Lynch syndrome: a consensus statement by the US Multi-Society Task Force on colorectal cancer. Gastroenterology 2014;147(2):502–26.

increased and some FAP patients develop intra-abdominal desmoid tumors, which can be a significant source of morbidity and mortality.

Germline mutations in *adenomatous polyposis coli* (*APC*), a tumor suppressor gene that regulates beta catenin in Wnt signaling, can be identified in 90% of individuals with classic FAP. Somatic mutations in *APC* occur in up to 80% of all CRCs, and represent the first step in the adenoma-carcinoma transformation.[27] Germline *APC* mutations occur at a population frequency of 1 in 7000. *APC* is a very large gene (15 exons) and phenotypes can vary based on location of the mutation, and individuals with germline mutations in *APC* in 3′ and 5′ ends are more likely to have fewer polyps, which may develop at later ages. Although FAP is characterized by autosomal dominant transmission, up to 30% of *APC* mutation carriers have no family history of the disease and are believed to represent de novo mutations.

### Diagnosis

The diagnosis of FAP is usually made based on the extensive adenomatous polyposis of the colon, and genetic testing confirms germline *APC* mutations in 90% of individuals affected with the classic phenotype. Approximately 5% to 10% of germline *APC* mutations exhibit attenuated colonic polyposis phenotypes (10–100 adenomas); thus genetic evaluation should be considered for individuals with more than 10 to 20 adenomas.[23,28] The identification of mutations in other genes (eg, *MUTYH*, *POLE*, *POLD1*; see later discussion) in some individuals with adenomatous polyposis suggests diverse genetic causes for adenomatous polyposis and there additional genes may yet be discovered.

### Management

The risk for CRC associated with classic adenomatous polyposis is very high, requiring careful surveillance and/or prophylactic surgery. The timing of surgery depends on the polyp burden. Colonoscopic surveillance in *APC* mutation carriers should begin at age 10 to 12 years and continue until polyp burden is no longer amenable to endoscopic control, at which time surgical colectomy would be indicated. Surgical options include total proctocolectomy with ileoanal anastomosis, ileorectal anastomosis, or end ileostomy. Surveillance of any remaining rectal tissue and/or ileal pouch should continue at 6 to 12 month intervals with the goal of removing all polyps.

Nearly half of FAP patients will develop clinically significant adenomas in their upper gastrointestinal tract; thus endoscopic surveillance (using a standard endoscope and duodenoscope) should be performed at intervals ranging from 6 month to 5 years depending on polyp burden.[29] Severity of duodenal disease can be assessed using the Spigelman stage,[30] and the goal of surveillance should be to remove any duodenal and/or ampullary adenomas that are large (>10 mm) or contain high-grade dysplasia. Because Spigelman stage IV duodenal polyposis is associated with high risk for malignant transformation, these individuals may be candidates for surgery (pancreas-sparing duodenectomy vs Whipple). Gastric polyps are common in individuals with FAP and some individuals develop extensive gastric polyposis, which is usually made up of fundic gland polyps. Although low-grade dysplasia is often reported in fundic gland polyps, this does not seem to be associated with malignant transformation. Gastric cancer is uncommon in FAP and gastric surgery should only be considered for patients with gastric cancer or gastric adenomas with high-grade dysplasia not amenable to endoscopic resection.

Chemoprevention agents can have a role in management of individuals who have undergone colectomy but still have significant polyp burden in the duodenum and/or rectum. Sulindac and cyclooxygenase (COX)-2 inhibitors have demonstrated some effectiveness; however, the occurrence of interval neoplasms in some individuals on long-term therapy emphasizes the importance of continued surveillance. Studies are ongoing to assess the effectiveness of these medications for controlling polyp burden in FAP patients who have not undergone colectomy; however, at this time, chemoprevention should not be considered as an equivalent alternative to colectomy.[23]

With regard to extraintestinal surveillance, given the increased risk for thyroid cancer thyroid screening (physical examination and/or ultrasound) should be considered for patients with FAP. Desmoid tumors can be a significant source of morbidity for some patients and, because management of these neoplasms can be challenging, consultation with expert centers can be of value.

### MUTYH-Associated Polyposis

Some individuals presenting with classic polyposis without a detectable *APC* mutations have been found to carry biallelic mutations in *MUTYH*, a base excision repair gene.[31] *MUTYH*-associated polyposis (MAP) has since been associated with a variety of clinical phenotypes, including autosomal recessive polyposis, attenuated polyposis, and even CRCs developing in the absence of polyps. Population-based studies have identified monoallelic mutations at a population frequency of 1 in 100, with biallelic *MUTYH* mutations in 1.7% of unselected CRC cases.[32] Although some individuals with biallelic *MUTYH* mutations have colonic and extracolonic features that resemble classic FAP, most individuals with MAP manifest attenuated polyposis, frequently with fewer than 20 adenomas.

Colorectal surveillance for individuals with MAP involves colonoscopy every 1 to 2 years, with the interval dictated largely by the polyp burden. Because some individuals can develop polyps of the upper gastrointestinal tract, a baseline upper endoscopy should be considered.[23]

### Polymerase Proofreading Associated Polyposis

Polymerase proofreading–associated polyposis (PPAP) is associated with germline mutations in *POLE* and *POLD1*, which were originally identified as somatic mutations in hypermutated CRC tumors.[33] Germline mutations in *POLE* and *POLD1* have been identified in rare families with highly penetrant autosomal dominant CRC.[34] The clinical phenotype of PPAP families is variable and, although the original families were characterized by multiple individuals affected with multiple colorectal adenomas, germline mutations have been found in families with a nonpolyposis phenotype. In addition, *POLE* and *POLD1* germline mutations have been associated with increased risks for endometrial cancer[35] and duodenal cancer.[36] At this time, cancer surveillance is dictated by clinical phenotype.

### Hamartomatous Polyposis Syndromes

Hamartomatous polyposis, defined as occurrence of more than 3 to 5 hamartomatous polyps in the gastrointestinal tract, is rare, implicated in less than 0.5% of all CRC cases.[4] Germline mutations in *SMAD4 and BMPR1A* (juvenile polyposis syndrome [JPS]), *STK11* (Peutz-Jeghers syndrome [PJS]), and *PTEN* (PTEN hamartoma tumor syndrome [PHTS] or Cowden syndrome) predispose to development of hamartomatous polyps as well as various gastrointestinal and other associated cancers.

### Juvenile polyposis syndrome

JPS, which often presents with multiple hamartomatous polyps in the stomach and/or colon, is associated with germline mutations in *SMAD4* and *BMPR1A*, which encode proteins involved in the transforming growth factor beta signaling pathway. JPS-associated hamartomatous polyps can be associated with symptomatic gastrointestinal blood loss and potential for malignant transformation. Although most patients can be managed endoscopically with upper and lower endoscopy at 1 to 3 year intervals, surgical colectomy and/or gastrectomy is sometimes warranted. *SMAD4* mutations are associated with risk for hereditary hemorrhagic telangiectasia, and mutation carriers should be screened for cerebrovascular and pulmonary arteriovenous malformations.[23]

### Peutz-Jeghers syndrome

PJS, is characterized by multiple hamartomatous gastrointestinal polyps, mucocutaneous pigmentation, and increased risk for cancers of multiple types. Small bowel hamartomas can result in intussusception and small bowel obstruction, a common clinical presentation. Germline mutations in *STK11* are identified in 50% to 70% of affected individuals and are associated with increased risk for gastrointestinal tumors (gastric, colorectal, pancreatic), as well as breast, genitourinary, and lung cancers, with estimated lifetime risk for developing any cancer ranging from 37% to 93%.[37,38]

Recommended surveillance for individuals with PJS includes screening for small bowel polyps (with video capsule endoscopy or MR enterography), upper endoscopy, and colonoscopy at 1 to 3 year intervals, depending on polyp burden. The high risk for extraintestinal cancers warrants enhanced surveillance for breast cancer (MRI and mammogram beginning at age 25 years) and gynecologic tumors (pelvic examination and transvaginal ultrasound). Because of the high lifetime risk for pancreatic cancer, it is reasonable to begin screening with MR cholangiopancreatography and/or endoscopic ultrasound at age 35 years.[23]

### Cowden syndrome

Cowden syndrome (or PHTS) is associated with germline mutations the phosphatase and tensin homolog (*PTEN*). The clinical phenotype of germline mutation carriers is highly variable and includes increased risk for many different cancer types (notably breast, thyroid, endometrial, and kidney)[39] as well as characteristic physical examination findings (macrocephaly, oral mucosal cobblestoning, pigmentation of the glans penis, cutaneous trichilemmoma, and multiple lipoma). The gastrointestinal phenotype can be variable as well, with the colonic phenotype ranging from no polyps to multiple gastrointestinal hamartomas, adenomas, serrated polyps, hyperplastic polyps, and ganglioneuromas; and the degree to which risk for CRC may be increased likely depends on the individual's phenotype.[40] *PTEN* mutation carriers can develop upper gastrointestinal tract findings, including gastroduodenal polyps and esophageal acanthosis glycans. Gastrointestinal tract surveillance includes upper endoscopy and colonoscopy every 1 to 3 years depending, on polyp burden. The high risk for extraintestinal cancers requires enhanced breast surveillance, as well as screening for uterine, thyroid, and kidney cancers.

### Serrated Polyposis

Serrated polyposis (previously known as hyperplastic polyposis) has been defined by the World Health Organization based on any of the following[41]: (1) 5 or more serrated polyps proximal to the sigmoid colon with at least 2 measuring greater than 10 mm, (2) any number of serrated polyps in the proximal colon in an individual who has a first-degree relative with serrated polyposis, or (3) greater than 20 serrated polyps of any size distributed throughout the colon. Sessile serrated polyps are thought to be the precursors of CRCs that arise through the serrated pathway of colorectal neoplasia,[42,43] most of which exhibit DNA MMR deficiency phenotypes or MSI with loss of protein expression of MLH1 and PMS2. The heterogeneity among cases and the lack of an identifiable genetic cause raise concerns that serrated polyposis may not be a single disease.[44] Although biallelic *MUTYH* mutations have been reported in some individuals meeting criteria for serrated polyposis,[45] clinical genetic testing is rarely informative.

Colonoscopy with polypectomy is the recommended management strategy for serrated polyposis; however, these polyps can be difficult to visualize and some studies suggest these lesions may be more likely to progress to cancers when compared with conventional adenomas[46] and lifetime CRC risk estimates range from 7% to 50%.[47,48] Consequently, colonoscopy every 1 to 3 years is required, with consideration of surgical colectomy for patients whose polyp burden is not amenable to endoscopic control.

### Familial Colorectal Cancer Type X

Approximately 40% to 50% of families with what seems to be autosomal dominant CRC meeting Amsterdam criteria have tumors that are DNA MMR proficient and do not have detectable germline mutations in DNA MMR genes. This subgroup of HNPCC is referred to as familial CRC type X (FCCX).[49] Despite extensive efforts to identify germline mutations in FCCTX families, a single unifying genetic diagnosis has not been identified. In contrast to Lynch syndrome, in FCCTX the average age at CRC diagnosis is older, and risk for CRC seems to be only moderately (2-fold to 3-fold) higher than general population risk, without increase in risk for extracolonic tumors.[49,50] Consequently, cancer surveillance is much less intense for FCCTX families than for Lynch syndrome, and colonoscopy every 3 to 5 years seems to be effective.

### Other Genetic Syndromes Associated with Colorectal Cancer Type Risk

There are genetic mutations associated with other hereditary syndromes that confer increased risk for CRC. Germline mutations in the *TP53* tumor suppressor gene associated with Li Fraumeni syndrome have been identified in 1.3% of individuals with young onset CRC[51] and 1% to 2% of patients undergoing genetic testing for suspected Lynch syndrome have been found to carry mutations in *BRCA1* and *BRCA2* associated with hereditary breast ovarian cancer syndrome.[52] Because next-generation sequencing technologies facilitate sequencing multiple genes simultaneously, use of multiplex gene panel testing offers opportunities to identify mutations in high and moderate penetrance cancer genes. Although use of multiplex gene panels has been shown to increase the number of pathogenic mutations identified in patients with breast[53] and ovarian[54] cancers, the clinical implications of germline mutations in genes associated with low or moderate cancer risks (eg, *CHEK2*, *ATM*) on CRC risk remain unclear.[55]

## GASTRIC CANCER

Although most gastric adenocarcinomas are presumed to be sporadic, approximately 5% to 10% arise in individuals with a family history of gastrointestinal cancer and it is estimated that 3% to 5% are associated germline mutations implicated in inherited cancer predisposition syndromes.[56] Gastric adenocarcinomas can be classified broadly into intestinal and diffuse (signet ring cell) subtypes. Intestinal-type gastric cancers have been associated with several hereditary cancer syndromes, including

Lynch syndrome, PJS,[38] JPS,[56] FAP, hereditary breast and ovarian cancer,[57] and Li Fraumeni syndrome.[58]

Diffuse gastric cancers are much less common than intestinal cancers, and make up only 10% to 15% of gastric cancers. Unlike intestinal cancers, which typically present as a mass or ulcer, diffuse gastric cancers can be difficult to diagnose endoscopically and frequently present with linitis plastica and/or submucosal infiltrating signet ring cells. Diffuse gastric cancers are associated with mutations in the tumor suppressor gene E-cadherin or *CDH1* and the identification of a germline mutation in *CDH1* has significant implications for treatment of patients who have gastric cancer and their at-risk family members.

### Hereditary Diffuse Gastric Cancer

Hereditary diffuse gastric cancer (HDGC) is defined clinically as 2 or more cases of diffuse gastric cancer with 1 individual diagnosed at age less than 50 years or 3 or more cases of diffuse gastric cancer regardless of age.[59] Germline mutations in *CDH1* are identified in approximately half of families meeting these criteria and are associated with lifetime risk for gastric cancer of 40% to 60%.[59] Women with *CDH1* mutations have a lifetime risk for developing lobular breast cancer of 40% to 60%.

#### Diagnosis

The clinical spectrum of disease associated with *CDH1* mutations can vary. Whereas historically the diagnosis required cases of diffuse gastric cancer in multiple relatives, disease penetrance and expressivity can vary and revised guidelines have expanded indications for genetic testing. Genetic evaluation should be considered for any individual with a diagnosis of signet ring cell gastric cancer, bilateral lobular breast cancer at age less than 50 years, or with relatives affected with diffuse gastric cancer and/or lobular breast cancer diagnosed at age less than 50 years (**Box 3**).[60]

#### Management

Identification of a germline *CDH1* mutation has significant implications for management for cancer-affected patients and at-risk family members. Because *CDH1*-associated gastric cancers are characterized by submucosal spread, individuals

---

**Box 3**
**Clinical criteria for genetic testing for hereditary diffuse gastric cancer (CDH1)**

*Established criteria*

1. Two gastric cancer cases in the family: 1 confirmed diffuse type

2. Diffuse gastric cancer diagnosed at age less than 40 years

3. Personal or family history (first-degree or second-degree relative) of diffuse gastric cancer and lobular breast cancer, 1 diagnosed at age less than 50 years

*Testing could be considered*

1. Bilateral lobular breast cancer, or 2 cases of lobular breast cancer diagnosed age less than 50 years

2. Personal or family history of cleft lip or palate and family history of diffuse gastric cancer

3. In situ signet ring cells or pagetoid spread of signet ring cells

*From* van der Post RS, Vogelaar IP, Carneiro F, et al. Hereditary diffuse gastric cancer: updated clinical guidelines with an emphasis on germline CDH1 mutation carriers. J Med Genet 2015;52:361–74; with permission.

diagnosed with diffuse gastric cancer should undergo total gastrectomy. Furthermore, given the high lifetime risk for gastric cancer and limited sensitivity of endoscopic surveillance, presymptomatic CDH1 mutation carriers should be advised to undergo prophylactic total gastrectomy. Patients who opt not to undergo prophylactic gastrectomy should be advised to continue endoscopic surveillance; however, it is not uncommon for cancers to be diagnosed in individuals under endoscopic surveillance[61] and foci of signet ring cells are often identified in gastrectomy specimens following normal endoscopy examinations.[62] Consequently, guidelines recommend that *CDH1* mutation carriers undergo prophylactic total gastrectomy in early adulthood.[59,60] Given the high risk for lobular breast cancer, *CDH1* mutation carriers require enhanced breast cancer surveillance with MRI and mammogram similar to what is recommended for *BRCA1* and *BRCA2* mutation carriers.[56]

## PANCREATIC ADENOCARCINOMA

Although most pancreatic cancers are believed to be sporadic, approximately 10% of patients who have pancreatic cancer have 1 or more affected relatives, meeting criteria for familial pancreas cancer. Risk for pancreatic cancer can be seen in association with several known hereditary cancer syndromes. Individuals with hereditary breast ovarian cancer syndrome have a risk for pancreatic cancer, which is 2-fold to 4-fold higher compared with the general population, and a recent study identified germline mutations in *BRCA1* or *BRCA2* in 4.6% of unselected patients who have pancreatic cancer.[63] Risk for pancreatic cancer is similarly increased for individuals with Lynch syndrome.[64] Mutations in *CDKN2A*, associated with familial atypical mole multiple melanoma syndrome are associated with a lifetime risk for pancreatic cancer of 20% to 30%.[65] Individuals with PJS (*STK11*) are at very high risk for pancreatic cancer, with a relative risk of 132.[37] Germline mutations in the cationic trypsinogen gene *(PRSS1)* associated with hereditary pancreatitis have also been associated with lifetime risk for pancreatic cancer of up to 40%. Consequently, obtaining a family history that includes cancers of different types (breast, ovarian, melanoma, other gastrointestinal), as well as pancreatitis, is important for genetic risk assessment.

Approximately 10% of patients diagnosed with pancreatic cancer meet criteria for familial pancreatic cancer and germline mutations are identified in approximately 10% of these families, with mutations in *BRCA2* and *BRCA1* as the most common finding, followed by *CDKN2A* and *PALB2*.[66] Although recent reports have found germline variants in *ATM* overrepresented among familial pancreatic cancer families, the magnitude of cancer risk associated with *ATM* mutations has not yet been well defined.[67]

### Diagnosis

Although 90% of familial pancreatic cancer cases have no identifiable germline mutations, clinical genetics evaluation should be considered for individuals with multiple relatives affected with pancreatic cancer meeting criteria for familial pancreatic cancer,[23] as well as those reporting family histories in which there is an excess of associated cancers (eg, breast, ovarian, melanoma, colorectal) suggestive of possible inherited predisposition.

### Management

Identification of a germline alteration in a gene involved in DNA repair (eg, *BRCA2*, *BRCA1*, and *PALB2*) has important treatment implications for patients who have pancreatic cancer. Poly(ADP)-ribose polymerase inhibitor (PARPi) has been found to be effective in treatment of certain cancers that arise in the setting of defective function of homologous recombination DNA repair pathways.[68] Consequently, patients with pancreatic adenocarcinomas with loss of function of BRCA1, BRCA2, or PALB2 (either as a result of germline or somatic mutations) may be candidates for treatment with PARPi.

There are currently insufficient data to demonstrate that pancreatic cancer screening is effective in reducing morbidity and mortality from pancreatic cancer. However, guidelines from the International Cancer of the Pancreas Screening consortium recommend that screening be considered for high-risk individuals who meet specific criteria (**Box 4**), alternating endoscopic ultrasound and MRI, with the goal of early identification of neoplasms amenable to surgical resection.[69]

## CLINICAL APPROACH TO GENETIC RISK ASSESSMENT FOR GASTROINTESTINAL CANCER RISK

In caring for patients with and without a cancer diagnosis, clinicians are expected to make an assessment about whether or not there is concern for a heritable cancer syndrome.[70] To do this, the clinician must elicit a family history that (1) includes all cancer diagnoses in a patient's first-degree and second-degree relatives and (2) is sufficiently comprehensive to make an assessment about the possibility of a genetic diagnosis. Consequently, it is important to facilitate collection of detailed family history information and integrate it into electronic health record systems for use at point-of-care in outpatient clinics, endoscopy units, or inpatient settings. Incorporation of validated genetic risk models (BRCAPro, MMRPro, PREMMM1,2,6) and clinical diagnostic algorithms into electronic decision-support systems can help identify individuals whose risk of germline mutation meets the threshold for which genetic testing is recommended. Screening tumors for histopathology and/or molecular features associated with hereditary cancer syndromes (eg, DNA MMR deficiency for colon cancers, presence of signet ring cell histology in gastric cancers, somatic BRCA1 or BRCA2 mutations in

---

**Box 4**
**International Cancer of the Pancreas Screening consortium consensus summary on who should be considered for pancreatic cancer screening**

1. Individuals with 3 or more blood relatives affected with pancreatic cancer, with at least 1 affected FDR

2. Individuals with at least 2 affected FDRs with pancreatic cancer, with at least 1 affected FDR

3. Individuals with 2 or more affected blood relatives with pancreatic cancer, with at least 1 affected FDR

4. All patients with PJS syndrome should be screened, regardless of family history of pancreatic cancer.

5. CDKN2A/p16 carriers with 1 affected FDR

6. BRCA2 mutation carriers with 1 affected FDR (or 2 affected family members (no FDR) with pancreatic cancer

7. PALB2 mutation carriers with 1 affected FDR

8. MMR gene mutation carriers (Lynch syndrome) with 1 affected FDR

*Abbreviation:* FDR, first degree relative.

*From* Canto MI, Harinck F, Hruban RH, et al. International Cancer of the Pancreas Screening (CAPS) Consortium summit on the management of patients with increased risk for familial pancreatic cancer. Gut 2013;62(3):339–47; with permission.

pancreatic cancers) will also facilitate identification of individuals whose cancers developed in the setting of genetic predisposition.

Making the diagnosis of a hereditary cancer syndrome has an impact on management for patients who have cancer and their relatives. For the patient who has cancer, a genetic diagnosis can affect surgical approaches (eg, recommendation for subtotal colectomy in Lynch syndrome CRCs, total gastrectomy in HDGC), cancer therapeutics (eg, recommendation for PARPi for *BRCA* and *PALB2*-associated pancreatic cancer), as well as future cancer surveillance (eg, colonoscopy intervals in Lynch syndrome).

Genetic evaluation and interpretation of genetic test results can be complex. Determining the clinical significance of variants of uncertain significance in genes associated with known hereditary cancer syndromes and/or mutations in genes associated with moderate cancer risk is often not straightforward. Consequently, society guidelines recommend that genetic testing for hereditary cancer syndromes be performed in conjunction with before and after test counseling by providers with expertise in genetic testing.[71] Because cancer risks for individuals with hereditary cancer syndromes can involve multiple organ systems, management often requires coordination among multidisciplinary care teams. Integrating personal and family history along with tumor genomic features can facilitate early identification of individuals with genetic predisposition to cancer, expanding opportunities for treatment of patients who have cancer and for cancer prevention in their at-risk relatives.

## REFERENCES

1. Vogelstein B, Papadopoulos N, Velculescu VE, et al. Cancer genome landscapes. Science 2013;339:1546–58.
2. Evaluation of Genomic Applications in Practice and Prevention (EGAPP) Working Group. Recommendations from the EGAPP Working Group: genetic testing strategies in newly diagnosed individuals with colorectal cancer aimed at reducing morbidity and mortality from Lynch syndrome in relatives. Genet Med 2009;11:35–41.
3. Levin B, Lieberman DA, McFarland B, et al. Screening and surveillance for the early detection of colorectal cancer and adenomatous polyps, 2008: a joint guideline from the American Cancer Society, the US Multi-Society Task Force on Colorectal Cancer, and the American College of Radiology. Gastroenterology 2008;134:1570–95.
4. Jasperson KW, Tuohy TM, Neklason DW, et al. Hereditary and familial colon cancer. Gastroenterology 2010;138:2044–58.
5. NCCN. Genetic/Familial High-Risk Assessment: colorectal. NCCN Clinical Practice Guidelines in Oncology 2015. v. 2.2015. Available at: nccn.org. Accessed February 10, 2016.
6. Siegel RL, Jemal A, Ward EM. Increase in incidence of colorectal cancer among young men and women in the United States. Cancer Epidemiol Biomarkers Prev 2009;18:1695–8.
7. Mork ME, You YN, Ying J, et al. High prevalence of hereditary cancer syndromes in adolescents and young adults with colorectal cancer. J Clin Oncol 2015;33:3544–9.
8. Vasen HF, Mecklin JP, Khan PM, et al. The International Collaborative Group on Hereditary Non-Polyposis Colorectal Cancer (ICG-HNPCC). Dis Colon Rectum 1991;34:424–5.
9. Hampel H, Frankel WL, Martin E, et al. Screening for the Lynch syndrome (hereditary nonpolyposis colorectal cancer). N Engl J Med 2005;352:1851–60.

10. Hampel H, Frankel WL, Martin E, et al. Feasibility of screening for Lynch syndrome among patients with colorectal cancer. J Clin Oncol 2008;26:5783–8.

11. Fearon ER, Carethers JM. Molecular subtyping of colorectal cancer: time to explore both intertumoral and intratumoral heterogeneity to evaluate patient outcome. Gastroenterology 2015;148:10–3.

12. Chen S, Wang W, Lee S, et al. Prediction of germline mutations and cancer risk in the Lynch syndrome. JAMA 2006;296:1479–87.

13. Quehenberger F, Vasen HF, van Houwelingen HC. Risk of colorectal and endometrial cancer for carriers of mutations of the hMLH1 and hMSH2 gene: correction for ascertainment. J Med Genet 2005;42:491–6.

14. Jenkins MA, Baglietto L, Dowty JG, et al. Cancer risks for mismatch repair gene mutation carriers: a population-based early onset case-family study. Clin Gastroenterol Hepatol 2006;4:489–98.

15. Stoffel E, Mukherjee B, Raymond VM, et al. Calculation of risk of colorectal and endometrial cancer among patients with Lynch syndrome. Gastroenterology 2009;137:1621–7.

16. Aarnio M, Sankila R, Pukkala E, et al. Cancer risk in mutation carriers of DNA-mismatch-repair genes. Int J Cancer 1999;81:214–8.

17. Bonadona V, Bonaiti B, Olschwang S, et al. Cancer risks associated with germline mutations in MLH1, MSH2, and MSH6 genes in Lynch syndrome. JAMA 2011; 305:2304–10.

18. Umar A, Boland CR, Terdiman JP, et al. Revised Bethesda Guidelines for hereditary nonpolyposis colorectal cancer (Lynch syndrome) and microsatellite instability. J Natl Cancer Inst 2004;96:261–8.

19. Kastrinos F, Steyerberg EW, Mercado R, et al. The PREMM(1,2,6) model predicts risk of MLH1, MSH2, and MSH6 germline mutations based on cancer history. Gastroenterology 2011;140:73–81.

20. Giardiello FM, Allen JI, Axilbund JE, et al. Guidelines on genetic evaluation and management of Lynch syndrome: a consensus statement by the US Multi-Society Task Force on Colorectal Cancer. Gastroenterology 2014;147:502–26.

21. Palomaki GE, McClain MR, Melillo S, et al. EGAPP supplementary evidence review: DNA testing strategies aimed at reducing morbidity and mortality from Lynch syndrome. Genet Med 2009;11:42–65.

22. Yurgelun MB, Goel A, Hornick JL, et al. Microsatellite instability and DNA mismatch repair protein deficiency in Lynch syndrome colorectal polyps. Cancer Prev Res 2012;5:574–82.

23. Syngal S, Brand RE, Church JM, et al. ACG clinical guideline: Genetic testing and management of hereditary gastrointestinal cancer syndromes. Am J Gastroenterol 2015;110:223–62 [quiz: 63].

24. Carethers JM, Smith EJ, Behling CA, et al. Use of 5-fluorouracil and survival in patients with microsatellite-unstable colorectal cancer. Gastroenterology 2004; 126:394–401.

25. Le DT, Uram JN, Wang H, et al. PD-1 blockade in tumors with mismatch-repair deficiency. N Engl J Med 2015;372:2509–20.

26. Sharaf RN, Myer P, Stave CD, et al. Uptake of genetic testing by relatives of Lynch syndrome probands: a systematic review. Clin Gastroenterol Hepatol 2013;11: 1093–100.

27. Fearon ER, Vogelstein B. A genetic model for colorectal tumorigenesis. Cell 1990; 61:759–67.

28. Grover S, Kastrinos F, Steyerberg EW, et al. Prevalence and phenotypes of APC and MUTYH mutations in patients with multiple colorectal adenomas. JAMA 2012; 308:485–92.
29. Balmana J, Domchek SM, Tutt A, et al. Stumbling blocks on the path to personalized medicine in breast cancer: the case of PARP inhibitors for BRCA1/2-associated cancers. Cancer Discov 2011;1:29–34.
30. Spigelman AD, Williams CB, Talbot IC, et al. Upper gastrointestinal cancer in patients with familial adenomatous polyposis. Lancet 1989;2:783–5.
31. Sieber OM, Lipton L, Crabtree M, et al. Multiple colorectal adenomas, classic adenomatous polyposis, and germ-line mutations in MYH. N Engl J Med 2003; 348:791–9.
32. Balaguer F, Castellvi-Bel S, Castells A, et al. Identification of MYH mutation carriers in colorectal cancer: a multicenter, case-control, population-based study. Clin Gastroenterol Hepatol 2007;5:379–87.
33. Cancer Genome Atlas Network. Comprehensive molecular characterization of human colon and rectal cancer. Nature 2012;487:330–7.
34. Palles C, Cazier JB, Howarth KM, et al. Germline mutations affecting the proofreading domains of POLE and POLD1 predispose to colorectal adenomas and carcinomas. Nat Genet 2013;45:136–44.
35. Briggs S, Tomlinson I. Germline and somatic polymerase epsilon and delta mutations define a new class of hypermutated colorectal and endometrial cancers. J Pathol 2013;230:148–53.
36. Spier I, Holzapfel S, Altmuller J, et al. Frequency and phenotypic spectrum of germline mutations in POLE and seven other polymerase genes in 266 patients with colorectal adenomas and carcinomas. Int J Cancer 2015;137(2):320–31.
37. Giardiello FM, Trimbath JD. Peutz-Jeghers syndrome and management recommendations. Clin Gastroenterol Hepatol 2006;4:408–15.
38. van Lier MG, Wagner A, Mathus-Vliegen EM, et al. High cancer risk in Peutz-Jeghers syndrome: a systematic review and surveillance recommendations. Am J Gastroenterol 2010;105:1258–64 [author reply: 1265].
39. Mester J, Eng C. Cowden syndrome: Recognizing and managing a not-so-rare hereditary cancer syndrome. J Surg Oncol 2015;111(1):125–30.
40. Heald B, Mester J, Rybicki L, et al. Frequent gastrointestinal polyps and colorectal adenocarcinomas in a prospective series of PTEN mutation carriers. Gastroenterology 2010;139:1927–33.
41. Snover DC, Ahnen D, Burt R, et al, editors. Serrated polyps of the colon and rectum and serrated polyposis. 4th edition. Lyon (France): IARC; 2010.
42. Leggett B, Whitehall V. Role of the serrated pathway in colorectal cancer pathogenesis. Gastroenterology 2010;138:2088–100.
43. Snover DC. Update on the serrated pathway to colorectal carcinoma. Hum Pathol 2011;42:1–10.
44. Kalady MF, Jarrar A, Leach B, et al. Defining phenotypes and cancer risk in hyperplastic polyposis syndrome. Dis Colon Rectum 2011;54:164–70.
45. Boparai KS, Dekker E, Van Eeden S, et al. Hyperplastic polyps and sessile serrated adenomas as a phenotypic expression of MYH-associated polyposis. Gastroenterology 2008;135:2014–8.
46. Terdiman JP, McQuaid KR. Surveillance guidelines should be updated to recognize the importance of serrated polyps. Gastroenterology 2010;139:1444–7.
47. Boparai KS, Mathus-Vliegen EM, Koornstra JJ, et al. Increased colorectal cancer risk during follow-up in patients with hyperplastic polyposis syndrome: a multicentre cohort study. Gut 2010;59:1094–100.

48. Rex DK, Ahnen DJ, Baron JA, et al. Serrated lesions of the colorectum: review and recommendations from an expert panel. Am J Gastroenterol 2012;107: 1315–29 [quiz: 1314].

49. Lindor NM, Rabe K, Petersen GM, et al. Lower cancer incidence in Amsterdam-I criteria families without mismatch repair deficiency: familial colorectal cancer type X. JAMA 2005;293:1979–85.

50. Llor X, Pons E, Xicola RM, et al. Differential features of colorectal cancers fulfilling Amsterdam criteria without involvement of the mutator pathway. Clin Cancer Res 2005;11:7304–10.

51. Yurgelun MB, Masciari S, Joshi VA, et al. Germline mutations in patients with early-onset colorectal cancer in the colon cancer family registry. JAMA Oncol 2015;1(2):214–21.

52. Yurgelun MB, Allen B, Kaldate RR, et al. Identification of a Variety of Mutations in Cancer Predisposition Genes in Patients With Suspected Lynch Syndrome. Gastroenterology 2015;149(3):604–13.e20.

53. Kurian AW, Hare EE, Mills MA, et al. Clinical evaluation of a multiple-gene sequencing panel for hereditary cancer risk assessment. J Clin Oncol 2014;32: 2001–9.

54. Walsh T, Casadei S, Lee MK, et al. Mutations in 12 genes for inherited ovarian, fallopian tube, and peritoneal carcinoma identified by massively parallel sequencing. Proc Natl Acad Sci U S A 2011;108:18032–7.

55. Domchek SM, Bradbury A, Garber JE, et al. Multiplex genetic testing for cancer susceptibility: out on the high wire without a net? J Clin Oncol 2013;31:1267–70.

56. Chun N, Ford JM. Genetic testing by cancer site: stomach. Cancer J 2012;18: 355–63.

57. Brose MS, Rebbeck TR, Calzone KA, et al. Cancer risk estimates for BRCA1 mutation carriers identified in a risk evaluation program. J Natl Cancer Inst 2002;94: 1365–72.

58. Masciari S, Dewanwala A, Stoffel EM, et al. Gastric cancer in individuals with Li-Fraumeni syndrome. Genet Med 2011;13:651–7.

59. Fitzgerald RC, Hardwick R, Huntsman D, et al. Hereditary diffuse gastric cancer: updated consensus guidelines for clinical management and directions for future research. J Med Genet 2010;47:436–44.

60. van der Post RS, Vogelaar IP, Carneiro F, et al. Hereditary diffuse gastric cancer: updated clinical guidelines with an emphasis on germline CDH1 mutation carriers. J Med Genet 2015;52:361–74.

61. Lim YC, di Pietro M, O'Donovan M, et al. Prospective cohort study assessing outcomes of patients from families fulfilling criteria for hereditary diffuse gastric cancer undergoing endoscopic surveillance. Gastrointest Endosc 2014;80:78–87.

62. Seevaratnam R, Coburn N, Cardoso R, et al. A systematic review of the indications for genetic testing and prophylactic gastrectomy among patients with hereditary diffuse gastric cancer. Gastric cancer 2012;15(Suppl 1):S153–63.

63. Holter S, Borgida A, Dodd A, et al. Germline BRCA mutations in a large clinic-based cohort of patients with pancreatic adenocarcinoma. J Clin Oncol 2015; 33:3124–9.

64. Kastrinos F, Mukherjee B, Tayob N, et al. Risk of pancreatic cancer in families with Lynch syndrome. JAMA 2009;302:1790–5.

65. Lynch HT, Fusaro RM, Lynch JF, et al. Pancreatic cancer and the FAMMM syndrome. Fam Cancer 2008;7:103–12.

66. Zhen DB, Rabe KG, Gallinger S, et al. BRCA1, BRCA2, PALB2, and CDKN2A mutations in familial pancreatic cancer: a PACGENE study. Genet Med 2015;17(7): 569–77.
67. Grant RC, Selander I, Connor AA, et al. Prevalence of germline mutations in cancer predisposition genes in patients with pancreatic cancer. Gastroenterology 2015;148(3):556–64.
68. Comen EA, Robson M. Inhibition of poly(ADP)-ribose polymerase as a therapeutic strategy for breast cancer. Oncology 2010;24:55–62.
69. Canto MI, Harinck F, Hruban RH, et al. International Cancer of the Pancreas Screening (CAPS) Consortium summit on the management of patients with increased risk for familial pancreatic cancer. Gut 2013;62:339–47.
70. Lu KH, Wood ME, Daniels M, et al. American Society of Clinical Oncology Expert Statement: collection and use of a cancer family history for oncology providers. J Clin Oncol 2014;32:833–40.
71. Robson ME, Storm CD, Weitzel J, et al, American Society of Clinical Oncology. American Society of Clinical Oncology policy statement update: genetic and genomic testing for cancer susceptibility. J Clin Oncol 2010;28:893–901.

# Molecular Detection of Gastrointestinal Neoplasia

## Innovations in Early Detection and Screening

Bradley W. Anderson, MD, David A. Ahlquist, MD*

## KEYWORDS

- Gastrointestinal cancer • Early detection • Screening • Molecular markers
- Blood testing • Stool testing

## KEY POINTS

- Gastrointestinal (GI) malignancies account for 40% of all cancer deaths globally, but most types remain unscreened.
- With recent technology advances, new molecular screening tools under development could open doors for early detection of all GI cancers.
- Adjunctive molecular tests also have potential to extend the reach of the endoscopist for greater accuracy in detecting GI neoplasms.

## INTRODUCTION

Globally, gastrointestinal (GI) malignancies account for roughly 40% of all cancer deaths.[1,2] In the United States, upper GI cancers kill twice as many as does colorectal cancer (CRC); but, unlike CRC, rates for cancers of the pancreas, liver, and esophagus are increasing.[3] This year, pancreatic cancer surpasses breast as the third most common cancer killer[4] and by 2020 passes CRC as the second most common.[5] By 2030, hepatoma may overtake CRC as the third deadliest cancer.[5] Currently, most upper GI cancers present symptomatically at a late stage and are among the most lethal cancers.[6] These alarming trends are calls for action.

Effective early detection methods are needed desperately. However, with a few exceptions,[7] screening for upper GI cancers in most countries has not been pursued because of the relatively low prevalence of cancers at individual sites and lack of cost-effective screening tools.

Disclosures: Mayo Clinic has licensed technology to Exact Sciences related to the commercialized stool DNA test Cologuard. As co-inventor of licensed technology, Dr D.A. Ahlquist shares royalties to Mayo Clinic according to institutional policy. Funding provided by Carol M. Gatton endowment.
Division of Gastroenterology & Hepatology, Mayo Clinic, Gonda Building E-9, 200 First Street SW, Rochester, MN 55905, USA
* Corresponding author.
*E-mail address:* ahlquist.david@mayo.edu

This overview briefly examines molecular approaches as potential screening solutions to the challenge of GI cancer. It summarizes the types of molecular markers being considered, gives examples of molecular tools under development, and appraises the future role of molecular methods for universal detection of GI cancers. Although there are obvious implications on downstream endoscopic evaluation and management, these important clinical aspects are not addressed.

## MECHANISMS, MEDIA, AND MARKERS

The concept of molecular screening is based on measurement of tumor-derived markers in readily accessible media. The promise of this approach lies in its ease for patients and potential to open doors for cost-effective screening of multiple GI cancers with a single test. Several key biological and technical elements must come together for molecular screening to be feasible. First, markers must reliably enter and remain in the target medium to be detectable at earliest cancer stage and, ideally, with precancer. Second, assays with sufficient technical sensitivity are needed to detect tumor markers in low abundance. And, third, highly discriminant markers must be identified that are positive when a GI neoplasm is present but otherwise remain negative, and such markers would ideally also predict the anatomic site of the primary GI tumor. Fueled by rapid technical advances, there is intense academic interest in this approach and increasing development by industry.

With GI cancers there exists the unique opportunity for noninvasive screening by marker detection either in blood or, because of their shared property of luminal exfoliation,[7] in stool. A central obstacle with blood testing has been the difficulty detecting earliest stage cancer and precancer. Tumor markers are detected readily from circulation with later stage cancer, but are often below detection limits with stage I cancers and precancers.[8,9] In contrast, CRC and precancerous polyps exfoliate molecular markers abundantly into stool.[8,10,11] A direct comparison between stool and plasma testing of DNA markers in paired samples showed substantially higher marker levels and diagnostic yield with stool than with plasma (**Fig. 1A**), which prompted a conceptual model suggesting that the biological mechanism of marker release by exfoliation favors early stage detection over that by vascular invasion (**Fig. 1B**).[8] It may be possible to overcome the biological constraints of limited vascular invasion in early stage disease by exploiting potential alternative mechanisms of marker entry into blood, such as by release of exosomes (nanovesicles emitted from surface of tumor cells and containing proteins, RNA, and DNA)[12] or phagocytosis by circulating macrophages, or simply by improved analytical sensitivity to detect the associated low plasma levels of tumor markers. With stool testing, it is unclear how effectively markers exfoliated from upper GI tumors can be recovered after traversing the digestive gauntlet. Model systems suggest that the small quantities of cells estimated to be shed from upper GI tumors can be detected in stool using sensitive techniques,[13] and pilot case-control studies have demonstrated that it is possible to detect tumor markers in stool from patients with known upper GI cancer.[14,15]

A comprehensive summary of specific candidate tumor markers is beyond the scope of this clinical review. The major classes of markers include intact tumor cells and cellular constituents including proteins, RNA, and DNA; each class has diagnostic advantages and disadvantages.

### Whole Tumor Cells

Intact tumor cells may be recovered from the circulation. Sophisticated sequencing and other assay methods are now available to determine the genomic makeup

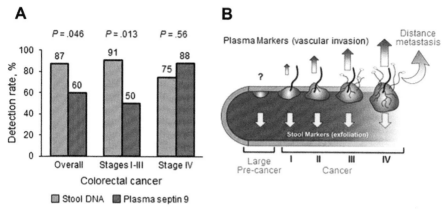

**Fig. 1.** Comparison of colorectal neoplasm detection by blood and stool testing for DNA markers. (*A*) Detection rates by multitarget stool DNA and plasma *septin 9* tests. Rates compared for overall group (n = 30), a subset without metastases (stages I-III; n = 22), and a subset with metastases (stage IV; n = 8). (*B*) Molecular marker release from colorectal neoplasms into target media. This conceptual model shows proportional differences (illustrated by *arrow* sizes) expected in rates of marker release into the bloodstream via the mechanism of vascular invasion and into the stool via the mechanism of exfoliation during progressive phases of tumorigenesis. Marker release into the bloodstream from precursor lesions is negligible but increases progressively with advancing stages of cancer. In contrast, marker release by exfoliation into stool occurs at comparable rates from large precancers and all stages of cancer. (*Adapted from* Ahlquist DA, Taylor WR, Mahoney DW, et al. The stool DNA test is more accurate than the plasma septin 9 test in detecting colorectal neoplasia. Clin Gastroenterol Hepatol 2012;10(3):272–7; with permission.)

(sometimes called "liquid biopsy"), which may obviate need for tumor biopsy in the future.[16] However, circulating tumor cells are undetectable generally with stage I cancer or precancer.[17,18] Tumor cells can also be recovered from stool but primarily with left-sided CRC and less with more proximal lesions.[19,20]

## Proteins

Classical protein markers, such as carcinoembryonic antigen,[21] carbohydrate antigen 19-9,[22] and alpha-1-antitrypsin,[23] have been helpful for prognosis and surveillance in colorectal, pancreatic, and liver cancers, respectively, but have failed in early detection.[23–25] Although proteins have the attractive features of test simplicity and low cost, many lack sufficient specificity or stability when assayed from distant media. Continued discovery efforts may yield discriminant marker candidates for future assays.

## RNA

Various RNA species may be overexpressed or underexpressed in neoplasms and potentially serve as early detection markers. An advantage over DNA-based markers is that there are several thousand RNA copies per cell, which could translate into greater sensitivity and a requisite for smaller sample size. A challenge with many RNA markers has been nonspecificity and nonreproducibility across studies.[26] Short RNA subtypes, such as microRNAs (miRNAs), may be more stable in stool or in blood.[27]

## DNA

The most studied class of tumor markers has been acquired DNA alterations, both genetic (eg, mutations, translocations) and epigenetic (eg, aberrant methylation). Important advantages of DNA markers include their distinguishing tumor-specific structural changes (rather than functional overexpression or underexpression, as occurs with protein or RNA) and relatively better stability.[28] A technical challenge in targeting acquired genetic changes relates to the large assay capacity required to achieve broad diagnostic coverage, often involving interrogation of thousands of potential mutation sites across multiple genes; continued progress in high-speed sequencing methods may allow a practical solution someday. In contrast, aberrant methylation typically occurs at the gene promoter region or other predictable single sites within a gene, and a small panel of methylated DNA markers may provide broad coverage.[29] Methylated DNA markers with site specificity have also been identified, a clinically relevant property that may allow the prediction of tumor location.[30]

## A GLIMPSE AT EMERGENT AND EXPERIMENTAL NEW MOLECULAR TOOLS FOR GASTROINTESTINAL CANCER SCREENING

New molecular tools may allow the accurate detection of both cancer and precancer at multiple GI sites, not only to create screening opportunities but to extend the diagnostic capabilities of the endoscopist as well.

### Esophageal Cancer

Esophageal cancer is the sixth leading cause of cancer mortality worldwide.[31] Esophageal adenocarcinoma predominates in Western countries and squamous cell carcinoma in Eastern countries. Incidence rates of both are increasing.[31] Both cancer types are highly lethal when presenting symptomatically, readily curable when detected at presymptomatic early stages, and preceded by recognizable precursor lesions.[32] Early studies have explored the feasibility of testing DNA markers in blood,[29–31] saliva,[32] and stool[10] for the screen detection and prognostic assessment of esophageal cancer.

#### Sponge-on-string device

A simple, ingestible sponge-on-string device (SOS) has emerged as a potential minimally invasive, accurate, and low-cost approach to the screen detection of Barrett's esophagus[33] (**Fig. 2**). Barrett's esophagus, the metaplastic precursor to adenocarcinoma, may be present in more than 5% of the US population[34]; current approaches to its detection and surveillance are endoscopic. The feasibility of SOS has been established when linked with an immune assay for trefoil factor 3 (a marker of intestinal metaplasia) on the recovered cytologic sample. In a case-control study, this approach yielded a sensitivity for Barrett's of 79.9% at a specificity of 92.4%; detection increased in proportion to Barrett's length.[35] Furthermore, modeling suggests that SOS is cost effective.[36] Alternative molecular markers may have merit with SOS, because preliminary data using novel methylated DNA markers detected 100% of Barrett's cases at 100% specificity (Iyer DDW 2016 abstract)[37]. By either SOS sampling or endoscopic brushing, use of molecular markers may also complement biopsy for detection of dysplasia during surveillance.[38] In a pilot study with a panel of methylated DNA markers applied to esophageal brushings, detection of Barrett's low- and high-grade dysplasias was 71% to 78% and of small stage I cancer was 100%.[39]

SOS may also have value in screening squamous cell carcinoma, a disease most prevalent in underserved Eastern populations. In a pilot study using SOS in Northern

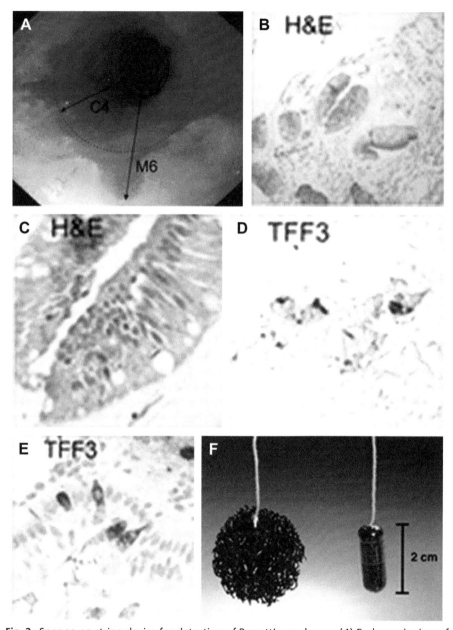

Fig. 2. Sponge-on-string device for detection of Barrett's esophagus. (*A*) Endoscopic view of Barrett's oesophagus. (*B*, *C*) Hematoxylin and eosin (H&E) and (*D*, *E*) trefoil factor 3 (TFF3) staining of Barrett's esophagus. (*F*) Cytosponge in gelatine capsule (*right*) and expanded (*left*). (*From* Kadri SR, Lao-Sirieix P, O'Donovan M, et al. Acceptability and accuracy of a non-endoscopic screening test for Barrett's oesophagus in primary care: cohort study. BMJ 2010;341:c4372; with permission.)

Iran, cytologic examination with p53 staining remarkably detected 100% of high-grade dysplasias at 100% specificity.[40]

## Gastric Cancer

Gastric cancer, the third most common cancer killer worldwide,[1] is often curable with pre-symptomatic early-stage detection but remains unscreened in most regions. Thus, there is a compelling rationale for noninvasive molecular screening. To date, no validated screening tests have been brought to practice. Investigators have explored miRNA and methylated DNA markers in blood,[41] and pilot DNA marker testing has suggested feasibility in stool as well.[10] For example, a recent study assessing the discrimination of a miRNA panel in plasma found moderate discrimination for stage I cancer with areas under the receiver operating characteristics curve of 0.99 and 0.081 in training and test sets, respectively.[42] Advances in whole methylome discovery have yielded highly accurate marker candidates with 100% sensitivity at 95% specificity (Anderson ACG 2015 abstract)[43]. Technical optimization and further rigorous clinical testing are needed.

### Gastric lavage
In a recent feasibility study,[44] assay of methylated DNA markers in simple gastric washings detected 90% of gastric cancer at 96% specificity. Further investigation of patient acceptance and accuracy with this approach are needed.

## Pancreatic Cancer

Most patients with pancreatic cancer present symptomatically at late stage. Its abysmal 5-year survival and alarming prevalence trend highlight the urgent need for improved early detection. Also, molecular tools may have adjunctive value for interrogation of the growing number of pancreatic cystic lesions incidentally found on abdominal imaging.

### Pancreatic juice
Pancreatic juice can be collected readily from the duodenum by standard upper endoscopy after stimulation of secretin. In a recent pilot study, an assay of novel methylated DNA markers from pancreatic juice accurately detected pancreatic cancer with an area under the receiver operating characteristics curve of 0.92[45]; distributions of a single marker, CD1D, in controls and cases with cancer are shown (**Fig. 3**). Optimization and further evaluation in larger studies are indicated.

### Cyst fluid
Management of pancreatic cysts represents a management conundrum, because most lesions are benign and structural features have proven inaccurate in predicting the presence of cancer or high-grade dysplasia.[46] Various molecular markers have been explored to improve the detection of advanced dysplasia in cysts.[47] A recent retrospective, multicenter study evaluated the combination of clinical features and DNA markers assayed from cyst fluid to detect lesions with mucinous features or dysplasia; cysts were accurately classified with a sensitivity of 90% to 100% and a specificity of 92% to 98%.[48] Others have explored miRNA markers for this diagnostic application.[49] Candidate methylated DNA markers have been identified able to discriminate high grade from low grade dysplasia in cysts with an area under the receiver operating characteristics curve of 0.91 [Majumder DDW 2016 abstract][50]; applied studies are under way.

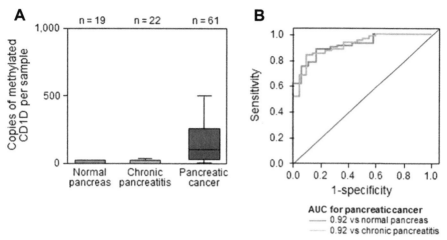

**Fig. 3.** Pancreatic cancer detection by endoscopically obtained pancreatic juice. (*A*) Copy numbers of methylated *CD1D* in pancreatic juice from patients with normal pancreas, chronic pancreatitis, and pancreatic cancer. (*B*) Receiver operating characteristics curves of methylated *CD1D* in pancreatic juice for the detection of pancreatic cancer in comparison to normal pancreas and chronic pancreatitis. AUC, area under the curve. (*From* Kisiel JB, Raimondo M, Taylor WR, et al. New DNA methylation markers for pancreatic cancer: discovery, tissue validation, and pilot testing in pancreatic juice. Clin Cancer Res 2015;21(19):4480; with permission.)

## Blood

Blood testing may play roles in both staging and screening. For staging pancreatic cancer, blood taken via endoscopic guidance from the portal vein seems to yield more tumor cells than from matched peripheral blood.[51] Circulating epithelial stem cells may also be present in blood with pancreatic cancer and even with premalignant cysts,[52] and may be a source for molecular interrogation. In a recent study, investigators found that miRNA panels differentiated pancreatic cancer cases from healthy and chronic pancreatitis controls using peripheral whole blood with areas under the curve ranging from 0.86 to 0.93; discrimination was superior to that of carbohydrate antigen 19-9.[53] Even higher discrimination for pancreatic cancer has been reported by serum assay of glypican-1 from circulating exosomes.[54] Further studies are needed to corroborate these interesting findings.

## Stool

Exploratory studies using nonoptimized markers and analytical methods have shown that pancreatic cancer can be detected by assay of exfoliated DNA markers in stool.[10,14] Further development has the potential to increase the detection rates with this noninvasive approach.

## Hepatobiliary Cancers

Worldwide, hepatoma represents the second major cancer killer.[55] Although cholangiocarcinoma constitutes only 2% of malignancies, it is the second most common primary hepatobiliary cancer.[56] There is a trend for rising incidence in the United States with both of these cancers.[55,56]

### Stricture brushing

The diagnostic evaluation of biliary strictures with conventional cytology obtained by endoscopic brushing has proved to be insensitive for detecting malignancy.[57] In a recent study on biliary stricture brushings, complementary use of fluorescent in situ hybridization improved cancer detection to 65% compared with only 18% by cytology alone.[58] Further improvements in diagnostic accuracy are needed. In a preliminary report, investigators assayed novel methylated DNA markers on archival brushings of biliary strictures and found a sensitivity of 100% at 90% specificity.[59]

### Cancer screening

Genome-wide methylation profiles have been described for hepatobiliary cancers at the tissue level[60–62] and have variably been explored in distant biological media. Methylated DNA markers for hepatoma detection have been assessed in plasma,[60] serum,[63] and peripheral blood mononuclear cells[64] with promising early results that suggest superiority over alpha fetoprotein levels. Candidate miRNA markers for hepatoma have been studied in plasma[65] and serum.[66] Pilot studies on molecular detection of hepatobiliary neoplasms have been reported using stool[15] and urine.[67]

## Colorectal Cancer

CRC is currently the second most common cause of cancer death in the United States.[68] Although screening reduces CRC mortality, conventional tools are variably accurate, associated with suboptimal compliance, and are not uniformly accessible. Innovative molecular approaches in stool or blood offer the promise of improved compliance and accessibility because of their noninvasive nature. Advances in molecular stool testing have recently led to a new commercial test with improved detection accuracy over fecal blood tests.

### Multitarget stool DNA test

Approved by both the Food and Drug Administration and the Centers for Medicare and Medicaid Services in 2014 as the first molecular screening test for CRC, the new multitarget stool DNA test (MT-sDNA) was included in the 2015 American Cancer Society CRC screening guidelines[69] and is now available for patient use (Cologuard, Exact Sciences, Madison, WI). A driver for the development of MT-sDNA was to improve participation rates based on its user-friendly features and ready access by mail. Early indicators seem to demonstrate success in this regard, because the test's manufacturer has publicly reported that 42% of the first 100,000 users disclosed on a questionnaire that this was their first CRC screen.

MT-sDNA targets a panel of exfoliated DNA markers (mutant KRAS plus 3 informative methylated genes, BMP3 and NDRG4) and hemoglobin. In an initial multicenter study using a prototype MT-sDNA, it was established that detection rates for CRC and advanced adenoma were not affected by lesion site.[70] Cutoffs for the optimized and automated MT-sDNA assay were established in a large case-control that which demonstrated sensitivities for CRC of 98% and for adenomas greater than 1 cm of 60% (72% for adenomas >2 cm, 83% for those >3 cm) at 90% specificity.[71] MT-sDNA performance was then validated in a 10,000-patient multicenter study from the screen setting using colonoscopy as the reference standard.[72] MT-sDNA detected 92% of CRC (94% for stages I and II) and 42% of advanced adenomas (66% for adenomas ≥2 cm) at a specificity of 90% (based on those with normal colonoscopy). For all lesion groups, detection rates by MT-sDNA exceeded those of fecal immunochemical test for occult blood (fecal immunochemical testing), although fecal immunochemical testing exhibited higher point specificity at 95%. A second cross-sectional screening study recently completed in Alaska Native people, who have among the world's highest CRC incidence rates,[73] showed MT-sDNA performance outcomes remarkably similar to those in the larger multicenter study[74] (**Fig. 4**).

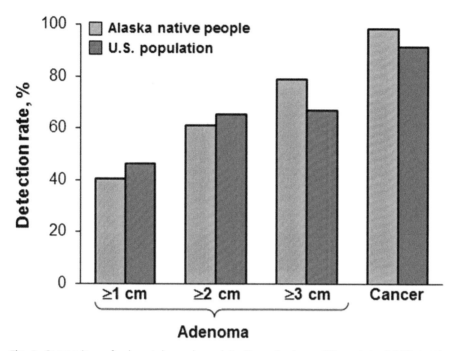

**Fig. 4.** Comparison of colorectal neoplasm detection rates by multitarget stool DNA test in Alaska Native people versus general US population. (*From* Redwood DG, Asay ED, Blake ID, et al. Stool DNA testing for screening detection of colorectal neoplasia in Alaska native people. Mayo Clin Proc 2016;91(1):6170; with permission.)

### Stool DNA testing for dysplasia surveillance in inflammatory bowel disease

Accurate molecular markers for dysplasia have potential value as adjuncts to colonoscopy in the surveillance of inflammatory bowel disease, a condition associated with increased CRC risk. In a pilot study using a panel of methylated DNA markers, stool DNA testing detected 100% of CRC and 80% of dysplasia.[75] Based on these encouraging early results, the test is being optimized and a multicenter study is underway.

### Blood

Numerous investigations are actively exploring different classes of markers in blood. A plasma test for methylated SEPTIN9 is available commercially for CRC screening but not yet approved by the Food and Drug Administration or included in screening guidelines. The SEPTIN9 test detects later stage CRC accurately, but has shown low sensitivity for stage I disease and fails to detect adenomas.[76] Similar findings were noted recently with plasma testing of alternative methylated DNA markers.[77] In contrast, a recent early study of selected miRNA markers assayed from circulating exosomes found stage I CRC detection rates greater than 90% at specificities greater than 90%,[78] and corroboration should be pursued.

### Universal Gastrointestinal Cancer Detection

Molecular technology allows the reimagination of the screening paradigm itself. Theoretically, a noninvasive blood or stool test could be used screen for all GI cancers from a conveniently singular sample. With such an approach, the entire GI tract could be functionally targeted as 1 organ, and the aggregate rather than single site tumor prevalence would be most relevant and, thereby, justify screening for tumors at all sites. Use of site-specific markers could direct the subsequent clinical evaluation to the likely location of the primary lesion to optimize efficiency. Indeed, exploratory studies suggest site prediction may be possible using miRNA[79] or methylated DNA[30,80] marker panels. Further technological advances and robust clinical validation studies are needed to actualize this vision.

## SUMMARY

Molecular approaches show promise for early detection across all major GI tumor types. However, many questions remain at this stage, and further research and development will be required to bring most of these new tools to practice.

## REFERENCES

1. Ferlay J, Soerjomataram I, Dikshit R, et al. Cancer incidence and mortality worldwide: sources, methods and major patterns in GLOBOCAN 2012. Int J Cancer 2015;136(5):E359–86.
2. Torre LA, Bray F, Siegel RL, et al. Global cancer statistics, 2012. CA Cancer J Clin 2015;65(2):87–108.
3. Simard EP, Ward EM, Siegel R, et al. Cancers with increasing incidence trends in the United States: 1999 through 2008. CA Cancer J Clin 2012;62(2):118–28.
4. Siegel RL, Miller KD, Jemal A. Cancer statistics, 2016. CA Cancer J Clin 2016; 66(1):7–30.
5. Rahib L, Smith BD, Aizenberg R, et al. Projecting cancer incidence and deaths to 2030: the unexpected burden of thyroid, liver, and pancreas cancers in the United States. Cancer Res 2014;74(11):2913–21.
6. Bowles MJ, Benjamin IS. ABC of the upper gastrointestinal tract: cancer of the stomach and pancreas. BMJ 2001;323(7326):1413–6.
7. Zou H. Pan-detection of gastrointestinal neoplasms by stool DNA testing: establishment of feasibility. Gastroenterology 2009;136:A625 [abstract: #T2036].
8. Ahlquist DA, Taylor WR, Mahoney DW, et al. The stool DNA test is more accurate than the plasma septin 9 test in detecting colorectal neoplasia. Clin Gastroenterol Hepatol 2012;10(3):272–7.e1.
9. Grutzmann R, Molnar B, Pilarsky C, et al. Sensitive detection of colorectal cancer in peripheral blood by septin 9 DNA methylation assay. PLoS One 2008;3(11): e3759.
10. Ahlquist DA. Next-generation stool DNA testing: expanding the scope. Gastroenterology 2009;136(7):2068–73.
11. Ahlquist DA, Harrington JJ, Burgart LJ, et al. Morphometric analysis of the "mucocellular layer" overlying colorectal cancer and normal mucosa: relevance to exfoliation and stool screening. Hum Pathol 2000;31(1):51–7.
12. Grasso L, Wyss R, Weidenauer L, et al. Molecular screening of cancer-derived exosomes by surface plasmon resonance spectroscopy. Anal Bioanal Chem 2015;407(18):5425–32.
13. Strauss BB, Yab TC, O'Connor HM, et al. Fecal recovery of ingested cellular DNA: implications for noninvasive detection of upper gastrointestinal neoplasms. Dig Dis Sci 2016;61(1):117–25.
14. Kisiel JB, Yab TC, Taylor WR, et al. Stool DNA testing for the detection of pancreatic cancer: assessment of methylation marker candidates. Cancer 2012; 118(10):2623–31.

15. Caldas C, Hahn SA, Hruban RH, et al. Detection of K-ras mutations in the stool of patients with pancreatic adenocarcinoma and pancreatic ductal hyperplasia. Cancer Res 1994;54(13):3568–73.
16. Karachaliou N, Mayo-de-Las-Casas C, Molina-Vila MA, et al. Real-time liquid biopsies become a reality in cancer treatment. Ann Transl Med 2015;3(3):36.
17. Bettegowda C, Sausen M, Leary RJ, et al. Detection of circulating tumor DNA in early- and late-stage human malignancies. Sci Transl Med 2014;6(224):224ra24.
18. Wong SC, Chan CM, Ma BB, et al. Clinical significance of cytokeratin 20-positive circulating tumor cells detected by a refined immunomagnetic enrichment assay in colorectal cancer patients. Clin Cancer Res 2009;15(3):1005–12.
19. Limburg PJ. Immunomagnetic isolation of malignant colonocytes from stool - Feasibility study in model system. Gastroenterology 1996;110(4):A551.
20. Koga Y, Yasunaga M, Moriya Y, et al. Detection of colorectal cancer cells from feces using quantitative real-time RT-PCR for colorectal cancer diagnosis. Cancer Sci 2008;99(10):1977–83.
21. Duffy MJ. Carcinoembryonic antigen as a marker for colorectal cancer: is it clinically useful? Clin Chem 2001;47(4):624–30.
22. Pavai S, Yap SF. The clinical significance of elevated levels of serum CA 19-9. Med J Malaysia 2003;58(5):667–72.
23. Hong WS, Hong SI. Clinical usefulness of alpha-1-antitrypsin in the diagnosis of hepatocellular carcinoma. J Korean Med Sci 1991;6(3):206–13.
24. Thomas DS, Fourkala EO, Apostolidou S, et al. Evaluation of serum CEA, CYFRA21-1 and CA125 for the early detection of colorectal cancer using longitudinal preclinical samples. Br J Cancer 2015;113(2):268–74.
25. Kim JE, Lee KT, Lee JK, et al. Clinical usefulness of carbohydrate antigen 19-9 as a screening test for pancreatic cancer in an asymptomatic population. J Gastroenterol Hepatol 2004;19(2):182–6.
26. Witwer KW. Circulating microRNA biomarker studies: pitfalls and potential solutions. Clin Chem 2015;61(1):56–63.
27. Etheridge A, Lee I, Hood L, et al. Extracellular microRNA: a new source of biomarkers. Mutat Res 2011;717(1–2):85–90.
28. Yang H, Xia BQ, Jiang B, et al. Diagnostic value of stool DNA testing for multiple markers of colorectal cancer and advanced adenoma: a meta-analysis. Can J Gastroenterol 2013;27(8):467–75.
29. Okugawa Y, Grady WM, Goel A. Epigenetic alterations in colorectal cancer: emerging biomarkers. Gastroenterology 2015;149(5):1204–25.e12.
30. Kisiel JB, Taylor WR, Yab TC, et al. Accurate site prediction of gastrointestinal cancer by novel methylated DNA markers: discovery & validation. Cancer Res 2015;75:4252.
31. Zhang Y. Epidemiology of esophageal cancer. World J Gastroenterol 2013; 19(34):5598–606.
32. Napier KJ, Scheerer M, Misra S. Esophageal cancer: a review of epidemiology, pathogenesis, staging workup and treatment modalities. World J Gastrointest Oncol 2014;6(5):112–20.
33. Kadri SR, Lao-Sirieix P, O'Donovan M, et al. Acceptability and accuracy of a non-endoscopic screening test for Barrett's oesophagus in primary care: cohort study. BMJ 2010;341:c4372.
34. Hayeck TJ, Kong CY, Spechler SJ, et al. The prevalence of Barrett's esophagus in the US: estimates from a simulation model confirmed by SEER data. Dis Esophagus 2010;23(6):451–7.

35. Ross-Innes CS, Debiram-Beecham I, O'Donovan M, et al. Evaluation of a minimally invasive cell sampling device coupled with assessment of trefoil factor 3 expression for diagnosing Barrett's esophagus: a multi-center case-control study. PLoS Med 2015;12(1):e1001780.

36. Benaglia T, Sharples LD, Fitzgerald RC, et al. Health benefits and cost effectiveness of endoscopic and nonendoscopic cytosponge screening for Barrett's esophagus. Gastroenterology 2013;144(1):62–73.e6.

37. Iyer P, Johnson ML, Lansing R, et al. Discovery, validation and feasibility testing of highly discriminant DNA methylation markers for detection of Barrett's esophagus using a capsule sponge device. Gastroenterol 2016;150(4):S66–7.

38. Fels Elliott DR, Fitzgerald RC. Molecular markers for Barrett's esophagus and its progression to cancer. Curr Opin Gastroenterol 2013;29(4):437–45.

39. Iyer PG. Detection of Barrett's dysplasia by assay of methylated DNA markers on whole esophageal brushings: a prospective feasibility study. Gastroenterology 2015;148(4):S-16.

40. Roshandel G, Merat S, Sotoudeh M, et al. Pilot study of cytological testing for oesophageal squamous cell dysplasia in a high-risk area in Northern Iran. Br J Cancer 2014;111(12):2235–41.

41. Jin Z, Jiang W, Wang L. Biomarkers for gastric cancer: Progression in early diagnosis and prognosis (Review). Oncol Lett 2015;9(4):1502–8.

42. Zhu C, Ren C, Han J, et al. A five-microRNA panel in plasma was identified as potential biomarker for early detection of gastric cancer. Br J Cancer 2014;110(9):2291–9.

43. Anderson BW, Suh Y, Choi B, et al. Gastric cancer detection by novel methylated DNA markers: Tissue validation in patient cohorts from the United States and South Korea. Am J Gastro 2015;110:S1033.

44. Watanabe Y, Kim HS, Castoro RJ, et al. Sensitive and specific detection of early gastric cancer with DNA methylation analysis of gastric washes. Gastroenterology 2009;136(7):2149–58.

45. Kisiel JB, Raimondo M, Taylor WR, et al. New DNA methylation markers for pancreatic cancer: discovery, tissue validation, and pilot testing in pancreatic juice. Clin Cancer Res 2015;21(19):4473–81.

46. Singhi AD, Zeh HJ, Brand RE, et al. American Gastroenterological Association guidelines are inaccurate in detecting pancreatic cysts with advanced neoplasia: a clinicopathologic study of 225 patients with supporting molecular data. Gastrointest Endosc 2016;83(6):1107–17.e2.

47. Jana T, Shroff J, Bhutani MS. Pancreatic cystic neoplasms: review of current knowledge, diagnostic challenges, and management options. J Carcinog 2015;14:3.

48. Springer S, Wang Y, Dal Molin M, et al. A combination of molecular markers and clinical features improve the classification of pancreatic cysts. Gastroenterology 2015;149(6):1501–10.

49. Wang J, Paris PL, Chen J, et al. Next generation sequencing of pancreatic cyst fluid microRNAs from low grade-benign and high grade-invasive lesions. Cancer Lett 2015;356(2 Pt B):404–9.

50. Majumder S, Taylor WR, Yab TC, et al. Detection of pancreatic high-grade dysplasia and cancer using novel methylated DNA markers: Discovery and tissue validation. Gastroenterol 2016;150(4):S120–121.

51. Catenacci DV, Chapman CG, Xu P, et al. Acquisition of portal venous circulating tumor cells from patients with pancreaticobiliary cancers by endoscopic ultrasound. Gastroenterology 2015;149(7):1794–803.e4.

52. Rhim AD, Thege FI, Santana SM, et al. Detection of circulating pancreas epithelial cells in patients with pancreatic cystic lesions. Gastroenterology 2014;146(3): 647–51.

53. Schultz NA, Dehlendorff C, Jensen BV, et al. MicroRNA biomarkers in whole blood for detection of pancreatic cancer. JAMA 2014;311(4):392–404.

54. Melo SA, Luecke LB, Kahlert C, et al. Glypican-1 identifies cancer exosomes and detects early pancreatic cancer. Nature 2015;523(7559):177–82.

55. Jemal A, Bray F, Center MM, et al. Global cancer statistics. CA Cancer J Clin 2011;61(2):69–90.

56. Blechacz BR, Gores GJ. Cholangiocarcinoma. Clin Liver Dis 2008;12(1):131–50.

57. Bowlus CL, Olson KA, Gershwin ME. Evaluation of indeterminate biliary strictures. Nature reviews. Gastroenterol Hepatol 2016;13(1):28–37.

58. Barr Fritcher EG, Voss JS, Brankley SM, et al. An optimized set of fluorescence in situ hybridization probes for detection of pancreatobiliary tract cancer in cytology brush samples. Gastroenterology 2015;149(7):1813–24.e1.

59. Ghoz HM. DNA methylation markers for detection of extrahepatic cholangiocarcinoma: discover, tissue validation, and pilot testing in biliary brush samples. Hepatology 2015;62(S1):295A.

60. Shen J, Wang S, Zhang YJ, et al. Genome-wide DNA methylation profiles in hepatocellular carcinoma. Hepatology 2012;55(6):1799–808.

61. Ammerpohl O, Pratschke J, Schafmayer C, et al. Distinct DNA methylation patterns in cirrhotic liver and hepatocellular carcinoma. Int J Cancer 2012;130(6): 1319–28.

62. Goeppert B, Konermann C, Schmidt CR, et al. Global alterations of DNA methylation in cholangiocarcinoma target the Wnt signaling pathway. Hepatology 2014; 59(2):544–54.

63. Hu L, Chen G, Yu H, et al. Clinicopathological significance of RASSF1A reduced expression and hypermethylation in hepatocellular carcinoma. Hepatol Int 2010; 4(1):423–32.

64. Zhang P, Wen X, Gu F, et al. Methylation profiling of serum DNA from hepatocellular carcinoma patients using an Infinium Human Methylation 450 BeadChip. Hepatol Int 2013;7(3):893–900.

65. Wen Y, Han J, Chen J, et al. Plasma miRNAs as early biomarkers for detecting hepatocellular carcinoma. Int J Cancer 2015;137(7):1679–90.

66. Lin XJ, Chong Y, Guo ZW, et al. A serum microRNA classifier for early detection of hepatocellular carcinoma: a multicentre, retrospective, longitudinal biomarker identification study with a nested case-control study. Lancet Oncol 2015;16(7): 804–15.

67. Chen S, Jain S, Lin S, et al. Development of a urine DNA based marker panel for early detection of liver cancer. Proceedings: AACR Annual Meeting 2014. San Diego (CA), April 5–9, 2014.

68. Haggar FA, Boushey R. Colorectal cancer epidemiology: incidence, mortality, survival, and risk factors. Clin Colon Rectal Surg 2009;22(4):191–7.

69. Smith RA, Manassaram-Baptiste D, Brooks D, et al. Cancer screening in the United States, 2015: a review of current American cancer society guidelines and current issues in cancer screening. CA Cancer J Clin 2015;65(1):30–54.

70. Ahlquist DA, Zou H, Domanico M, et al. Next-generation stool DNA test accurately detects colorectal cancer and large adenomas. Gastroenterology 2012; 142(2):248–56 [quiz: e25–6].

71. Lidgard GP, Domanico MJ, Bruinsma JJ, et al. Clinical performance of an automated stool DNA assay for detection of colorectal neoplasia. Clin Gastroenterol Hepatol 2013;11(10):1313–8.

72. Imperiale TF, Ransohoff DF, Itzkowitz SH. Multitarget stool DNA testing for colorectal-cancer screening. N Engl J Med 2014;371(2):187–8.

73. Kelly JJ, Alberts SR, Sacco F, et al. Colorectal cancer in Alaska native people, 2005-2009. Gastrointest Cancer Res 2012;5(5):149–54.

74. Redwood DG, Asay ED, Blake ID, et al. Stool DNA testing for screening detection of colorectal neoplasia in Alaska native people. Mayo Clin Proc 2016;91(1): 61–70.

75. Kisiel JB, Yab TC, Nazer Hussain FT, et al. Stool DNA testing for the detection of colorectal neoplasia in patients with inflammatory bowel disease. Aliment Pharmacol Ther 2013;37(5):546–54.

76. Lofton-Day C, Model F, Devos T, et al. DNA methylation biomarkers for blood-based colorectal cancer screening. Clin Chem 2008;54(2):414–23.

77. Pedersen SK, Symonds EL, Baker RT, et al. Evaluation of an assay for methylated BCAT1 and IKZF1 in plasma for detection of colorectal neoplasia. BMC Cancer 2015;15:654.

78. Ogata-Kawata H, Izumiya M, Kurioka D, et al. Circulating exosomal microRNAs as biomarkers of colon cancer. PLoS One 2014;9(4):e92921.

79. Rosenfeld N, Aharonov R, Meiri E, et al. MicroRNAs accurately identify cancer tissue origin. Nat Biotechnol 2008;26(4):462–9.

80. Nagasaka T, Tanaka N, Cullings HM, et al. Analysis of fecal DNA methylation to detect gastrointestinal neoplasia. J Natl Cancer Inst 2009;101(18):1244–58.

# The Role of the Microbiome in Gastrointestinal Cancer

Lydia E. Wroblewski, PhD[a], Richard M. Peek Jr, MD[a], Lori A. Coburn, MD[a,b],*

## KEYWORDS

- *Helicobacter pylori* • Gastric adenocarcinoma • Microbiota • Pyrosequencing
- Colon cancer • Inflammation

## KEY POINTS

- The risk of developing gastric cancer is multifactorial, and the microbiota has been identified as an important contributing factor.
- Colon cancer risk is modified by the gastrointestinal tract microbiota and environmental exposures, including diet, in addition to known genetic factors.
- With no single microbial causative agent identified, it is likely that an overall disturbance in the composition/metabolism of the colonic microbiota can promote cancer development.

## INTRODUCTION

In the last 2 decades, there has been a remarkable shift in identifying and understanding the multitude of microbes that colonize the human body. Previously, the *normal flora* was thought to be largely a silent passenger, only declaring itself when it traveled outside of its usual niche. However, it is now recognized that the microbiome, which is composed of bacteria, archaea, eukaryotes, and viruses, plays a key role in health and disease. Bacteria are the most abundant and well studied. The gastrointestinal (GI) microbiome is molded from birth by a multitude of interactions that can be distinct, such as the host genetic background, or variable, including diet, antibiotics, and other environmental exposures.[1,2]

Cancer is the second leading cause of death in the United States, and GI cancers represent a leading cause of morbidity and mortality.[3] Although genetic factors leading to an increased risk of cancer have been identified, such as adenomatous polyposis coli (*APC*) mutations that lead to familial adenomatous polyposis and

Disclosures/Conflict of Interest: The authors declare there are no conflicts of interest.
Sources of Funding: National Institutes of Health R01 DK58587, R01 CA77955, P01 CA116087, and P30 DK058404 to R.M.P. Department of Veterans Affairs 1IK2BX002126-01 to L.A.C.
[a] Division of Gastroenterology, Department of Medicine, Vanderbilt University School of Medicine, 2215 Garland Avenue, Nashville, TN 37232, USA; [b] Veterans Affairs Tennessee Valley Healthcare System, 1310 24th Avenue South, Nashville, TN 37212, USA
* Corresponding author. 2215 Garland Avenue, Suite 1030, Nashville, TN 37232.
*E-mail address:* lori.coburn@vanderbilt.edu

Gastroenterol Clin N Am 45 (2016) 543–556
http://dx.doi.org/10.1016/j.gtc.2016.04.010
0889-8553/16/$ – see front matter Published by Elsevier Inc.

**gastro.theclinics.com**

E-cadherin (*CDH1*) mutations that lead to hereditary diffuse-type gastric cancer (GC), these mutations do not account for most cases. In addition, the association of microbial infections with the risk for cancer development is well documented, including *Helicobacter pylori* with GC and hepatitis viruses with liver cancer.[4] Even nonpathogenic GI tract microbes, once considered inert, have been found to play a role in chronic inflammation, altering cell proliferation and stem cell dynamics, and altering immune surveillance mechanisms.[2,5] The focus of this review is the role of the GI microbiome in the development of gastric and colonic malignancies with a brief discussion of esophageal malignancy.

## GASTRIC CANCER

Gastric adenocarcinoma is the third leading cause of cancer-related death in the world.[6] In developed countries, the incidence of gastric adenocarcinoma has significantly decreased over the past century[7,8]; however, the incidence rates of both proximal gastric and gastroesophageal junction adenocarcinomas have increased in both the United States and Europe.[9,10] Chronic infection with *H pylori* is the strongest known risk factor for developing gastric adenocarcinoma.[11]

## HELICOBACTER PYLORI

*H pylori* is a gram-negative bacteria that selectively colonizes the gastric epithelium. Infection is usually acquired in childhood and, in the absence of combination antibiotic therapy, can persist for the lifetime of the host.[12] *H pylori* has colonized humans for almost 100,000 years[13]; approximately half of the world's population is infected with *H pylori*, promoting speculation that *H pylori* is an endogenous member of the gastric microbiota. Between 1% and 3% of *H pylori*–colonized persons develop gastric adenocarcinoma[14]; factors that play a role in the pathologic outcome of *H pylori* infection are varied, including strain-specific bacterial constituents; host genetic factors; environmental influences, including diet; and alterations in the host microbiota.[15]

## BACTERIAL AND HOST FACTORS AFFECTING THE PROPENSITY TOWARD GASTRIC CANCER

One *H pylori* virulence factor that influences GC risk is the *cag* pathogenicity island, which contains genes encoding proteins that form a type IV bacterial secretion system.[14] Another *H pylori* virulence factor linked to the development of GC is the secreted vacuolating cytotoxin A (VacA).[16,17] All *H pylori* strains contain *vacA*, but there are considerable differences in *vacA* sequences among strains. Strains containing type s1, i1, or m1 alleles within the 5′ region of the gene are highly associated with GC.[18–20] Host polymorphisms in interleukin (*IL*)-1$\beta$ and tumor necrosis factor (*TNF*)-$\alpha$ as well as environmental factors, such as a high-salt diet and low iron levels, in the context of *H pylori* infection also influence gastric carcinogenesis.[15]

Although *H pylori* infection is the strongest identified risk factor for developing GC, clinical trials suggest that other gastric microbiota constituents may influence disease progression. Antibiotic therapy directed against *H pylori* was reported to significantly decrease the incidence of GC in a 15-year follow-up study of 3365 subjects. Of note, more than 50% of the antibiotic-treated individuals remained colonized by *H pylori* at the 15-year follow-up.[21] These findings suggest that antibiotic treatment may attenuate the development of GC by inducing alterations in the non–*H pylori* microbiota.

## THE STOMACH MICROBIOTA IN GASTRIC PATHOGENESIS

The stomach harbors a large and diverse bacterial community ranging from $10^1$ to $10^3$ colony-forming units per gram,[22] which may influence gastric homeostasis and disease in conjunction with *H pylori* infection.[23]

The composition of the gastric microbiome in *H pylori*–negative individuals is highly diverse (**Fig. 1**). Sequencing of DNA isolated from human gastric biopsies identified 128 phylotypes within 8 bacterial phyla of which Proteobacteria, Firmicutes, Bacteroidetes, Fusobacteria, and Actinobacteria were the most abundant.[2,24] Using a newer technology, tagged 454 pyrosequencing, analysis of *H pylori*–negative biopsy samples identified 262 phylotypes representing 13 phyla.[25] These findings lend further support to the gastric microbiota being highly diverse, despite significant variability in the microbial composition between individuals.[24,25] In contrast, the microbiota among *H pylori*–infected individuals is much more uniform; *H pylori* represents the most abundant phylotype present in the stomach of *H pylori*–positive persons.[24,25] *H pylori* DNA accounted for 93% to 97% of all sequence reads in *H pylori*–positive persons and a total of 33 phylotypes were detected, more than 200 less than in *H pylori*–negative persons.[25] Taken together, these data suggest that *H pylori* colonization dramatically alters gastric microbiota diversity (see **Fig. 1**). Characterization of the human gastric microbiota using DNA microarrays detected 44 phyla with 4 dominant phyla: Proteobacteria, Firmicutes, Actinobacteria, and Bacteroidetes. Using this method, infection with *H pylori* was shown to increase the relative abundance of non–*H pylori* Proteobacteria, Spirochaetes, and Acidobacteria and decrease the relative abundance of Actinobacteria, Bacteroidetes, and Firmicutes compared with uninfected stomachs.[26] *H pylori* infection accounted for 28% of the variance in the microbiota; however, the bacterial communities in both *H pylori*–negative and –positive individuals remained highly complex.[26]

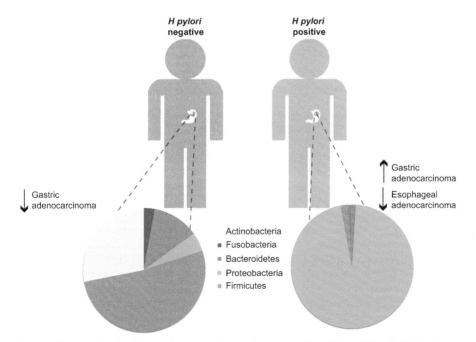

**Fig. 1.** The gastric microbiome in *H pylori*–negative versus *H pylori*–positive individuals.

Studies examining differences in microbial composition and outcomes of GC are more limited. Development of atrophic gastritis, which induces hypochlorhydria due to parietal cell loss, is a key step in the histologic progression to intestinal-type GC and can lead to overgrowth of non-*Helicobacter* microbiota, which may promote the progression towards GC.[27] Two recent studies have independently identified that proton pump inhibitor use may detrimentally alter the gut microbiota.[28,29]

When comparing the microbiota of 10 patients with GC to 5 dysplastic controls, the microbiota of patients with GC was found to be equally as diverse as dysplastic patients. Firmicutes, Bacteroidetes, Proteobacteria, Actinobacteria, and Fusobacteria were identified. The microbiota was predominately composed of species of *Streptococcus*, *Lactobacillus*, *Veillonella*, and *Prevotella*. *H pylori* were present in relatively low abundance.[30] More recently, pyrosequencing has been used to compare the gastric microbiota in persons with chronic gastritis, intestinal metaplasia, and GC. Pyrosequencing identified 10 bacterial phyla, and significant differences were observed in both the composition and diversity of the gastric microbiota in the histologic progression towards GC. Bacilli and members of the Streptococcaceae family were significantly enriched in GC samples compared with chronic gastritis and intestinal metaplasia samples, whereas Epsilonproteobacteria and Helicobacteraceae family members were decreased.[31]

An interesting new study compared the gastric microbiota of subjects from 2 Colombian populations: one at high-risk, Tuquerres, and one at low-risk, Tumaco, of developing GC. Despite high variability in the microbial composition between individuals, significant correlations were found with the town of origin.[32] Two operational taxonomic units, *Leptotrichia wadei*, which is associated with necrotizing enterocolitis and bacteremia, and a *Veillonella sp*, were significantly more abundant in Tuquerres. In the low-risk region of Tumaco, 16 operational taxonomic units, including a *Staphylococcus sp*, which is considered a constituent of the normal human microbiota, were significantly more abundant.[32] These results provide a tantalizing opportunity to manipulate the microbiota of animal models to more closely represent the microbiota of either the high-risk or low-risk populations of Colombia and determine key players in cancer development.

## ANIMAL MODELS TO STUDY THE MICROBIOME AND GASTRIC CANCER

Inbred mice with defined genotypes are commonly used to model carcinogenesis; however, this can be limited by uncontrolled microbial diversity within mice despite identical genetic backgrounds.[33,34] To counter this, gnotobiotic mice allow for controlling the microbiome and adding back individual or collections of microorganisms.

Similar to humans, the most abundant phylotypes in the mouse stomach are Bacteroidetes, Firmicutes, Proteobacteria, and Actinobacteria[33]; infection of mice with *H pylori* can alter the gastric microbiota.[35] *H pylori* infection induces gastritis in mice, and following *H pylori* infection for 2 months the gastric microbiota in specific pathogen free (SPF) mice harbored reduced numbers of *Lactobacillus* species and increased bacterial diversity.[35] An independent study, however, found that both acute and chronic infection of SPF C57BL/6 mice with *H pylori* failed to cause significant shifts in the gastric microbial composition.[36] It is possible that the inherent gastric microbial diversity of SPF mice may play a role in the outcome of *H pylori* infection.

INS-GAS mice are genetically predisposed to GC, and chronic interaction between *H pylori* and the gastric microbiota was found to influence disease progression in this model.[37] In SPF INS-GAS mice, GC spontaneously developed.[38,39] However, in germfree (GF) INS-GAS mice, cancer was slower to develop.[37] Moreover, *H pylori*-infected

GF INS-GAS mice developed less severe lesions and were slower to progress to GI intraepithelial neoplasia than *H pylori*–infected SPF INS-GAS mice.[37] A detailed analysis using 454 sequencing of partial 16S ribosomal DNA amplicons revealed specific differences in phyla between *H pylori*–infected and uninfected SPF INS-GAS mice. *H pylori* colonization led to an expansion in the proportion of Firmicutes and decreased numbers of Bacteroidetes while causing an overall increase in species diversity.[37] In fact, only 3 species of commensal bacteria (ASF356 *Clostridium* species, ASF361 *Lactobacillus murinus*, and ASF519 *Bacteroides species*) were required to promote gastric neoplasia in *H pylori*–infected GF INS-GAS mice to the same extent as that reported in *H pylori*–infected SPF INS-GAS mice.[40]

## ESOPHAGEAL ADENOCARCINOMA AND THE MICROBIOME

The incidence of esophageal adenocarcinoma has been increasing rapidly in developed countries over the past 40 years; this coincides with a decreasing incidence of *H pylori* infection and GC, suggesting that gastric colonization with *H pylori* may be protective against esophageal adenocarcinoma.[41] This protection could reflect inhibition of acid secretion via enhanced production of IL-1β and TNF-α in response to *H pylori* or through loss of parietal cells in atrophic gastritis.[23] Alternatively, changes in the gastric microbiota resulting from the loss of *H pylori* may increase the risk for an individual to develop esophageal cancer (see **Fig. 1**).[23]

The esophageal microbiome is altered during inflammation and metaplasia. Using a 16S rRNA gene survey, 2 types of microbiota, termed type I and type II, were identified in the esophagus.[42] The type I microbiome was dominated by gram-positive bacteria and the genus *Streptococcus*, whereas the type II microbiome was composed of a higher percentage of gram-negative bacteria, with the phyla Bacteroidetes, Proteobacteria, Fusobacteria, and Spirochaetes being the most abundant. The type II microbiome correlated with the histologic presence of esophagitis and Barrett's esophagus, whereas the type I microbiome was associated with a histologically normal esophagus.[42]

In a recent study, 30 esophageal adenocarcinoma cases were compared with 39 control subjects using cultured biofilms. In control subjects, 56 species belonging to 19 genera were detected, whereas in esophageal adenocarcinoma, 73 species from 23 genera were identified. Despite finding more species in esophageal adenocarcinoma than controls, no statistical differences were reported.[43] These findings provide an important framework for more detailed future studies delineating the structure and function of the esophageal microbiome and disease.

## COLORECTAL CANCER

Colorectal cancer (CRC) is the third leading cause of cancer mortality in the United States, and the risk of CRC increases with age.[3] Most of the cases are sporadic; however, up to 25% of patients have a family history of CRC but no evidence of an identified inherited syndrome.[44] This finding underscores the complex interaction of multiple genetic and epigenetic events contributing to CRC pathogenesis. The initiation of CRC can be due to mutations in tumor-suppressor genes, such as *APC*, *catenin (cadherin-associated protein) beta 1*, tumor protein *p53*, and the oncogene *Kirsten rat sarcoma viral oncogene homolog*, leading to a growth advantage in colonic epithelial cells progressing to adenomas and cancer.[23,44,45] Although these genetic mutations have clearly been linked to CRC development, the steps leading to the accumulation of these mutations and other epigenetic changes are not fully known. In addition to genetic alterations, microbial and environmental factors, including diet and lifestyle, have been shown in recent studies to play a role in promoting CRC.[46,47]

## THE MICROBIOME IN PATIENTS WITH COLONIC POLYPS OR COLORECTAL CANCER

Similar to the stomach and esophagus, the colon plays host to a complex and diverse population of microorganisms. These microorganisms outnumber human somatic and germ cells by at least an order of magnitude, and the collective microbial genome contains 100 or greater times more genes than the human genome.[48] Most of the colonic microbiota is composed of Bacteroidetes and Firmicutes, though other components include Proteobacteria, Actinobacteria, and Fusobacteria.[23,49] An individual's colonic microbiota is determined by factors such as environmental exposures, diet, and host genetics, although the identification of specific genetic factors leading to alterations in the microbiota is in a nascent stage.[50]

Although the microbiome contributes to both immune system development and the release of key nutrients and energy from dietary intake, alterations in the microbiome related to chronic inflammation seem to play a role in promoting the increased risk of carcinogenesis seen in patients with inflammatory bowel disease.[51] There is also mounting evidence that the microbiome plays a role in sporadic CRC[52–59] (**Table 1**). Studies of the fecal microbiota in patients with either CRC or colonic polyps have shown decreased temporal stability, with increased diversity of the *Clostridium leptum* and *C coccoides* subgroups versus control subjects, although not between patients with CRC versus colonic polyps.[60] Studies assessing mucosa-associated bacteria showed that the predominant phyla in control patients were Firmicutes, Bacteroidetes, and Proteobacteria.[61] Although patients with adenoma had a lower relative abundance of Bacteroidetes and a higher abundance of Proteobacteria, there was a trend toward increased diversity in patients with adenomas versus those without adenomas.[61] When similar studies assessed mucosa-associated microbiota in paired samples from patients with CRC (ie, tumor tissue and adjacent nontumor tissue), *Coriobacteridae*, *Roseburia*, *Fusobacterium*, and *Faecalibacterium*, which are generally regarded as gut commensals, were overrepresented in tumor tissue samples.[62] Multiple studies have assessed both the luminal and mucosa-associated microbiota in controls, patients with adenoma, and/or patients with CRC.[63,64] However, no single microbial species has been identified as a causative agent leading to a working model that overall disturbances in the composition, diversity, or functional properties of the colonic microbiota dysregulate the balance between the epithelium and the immune system towards inflammation, dysplasia, and ultimately cancer.

## DIET AND MICROBIAL METABOLITES

Epidemiologic studies have consistently indicated that diets with increased red meat and fat content (ie, Western diet) increase CRC risk, whereas increased fiber intake is associated with decreased CRC risk.[65,66] This alteration in risk by dietary intake may be facilitated by the colonic microbiota, which, for example, promote health via metabolism of fiber to produce short-chain fatty acids (SCFA), such as acetate, propionate, and butyrate.[65] Butyrate is the preferred energy source of colonic enterocytes and, along with propionate, has been shown to downregulate proinflammatory cytokines, such as IL-6 and IL-12, in colonic macrophages.[67] In addition, butyrate and propionate can induce forkhead box P3 (FOXP3)$^+$ regulatory T cells to control intestinal inflammation, thereby maintaining intestinal homeostasis.[67,68] The antiinflammatory effects of SCFAs not only influence host cells but may also contribute to homeostasis of the gut microbiota.[67,68]

**Table 1**
**Alterations in human gastrointestinal microbiota in patients with colonic adenoma and colorectal cancer**

| Patients | Sample Site | Changes in Microbiota | Study (Author, Year, Reference No.) |
|---|---|---|---|
| 20 Controls, 20 patients with polypectomy, and 20 patients with CRC (all s/p resection) | Fecal samples (3 samples over a 3-mo period for 20 polypectomy, 20 patients with CRC, as well as 6 of the control patients) | There was reduced temporal stability and increased diversity for the microbiota of patients with CRC and patients with polyps. In addition, there was increased diversity of the *Clostridium leptum* and *C coccoides* subgroups vs control subjects. | Scanlan et al,[60] 2008 |
| 21 Patients with adenoma and 23 controls | Rectal mucosal biopsies | Patients with adenoma had a trend toward increased diversity and richness vs controls. There was lower relative abundance of Bacteroidetes and higher abundance of Proteobacteria. | Shen et al,[61] 2010 |
| 6 Patients with CRC | Paired biopsies from tumor and adjacent nontumor tissue in the surgical resection specimen | The tumor areas had overrepresentation of *Coriobacteridae, Roseburia, Fusobacterium,* and *Faecalibacterium* and underrepresentation of Firmicutes and Enterobacteriaceae. | Marchesi et al,[62] 2011 |
| 46 Patients with CRC and 56 controls | Fecal samples; rectal swab samples; and from the patients with CRC, 27 with paired tumor and adjacent nontumor tissue | Overall the microbiota was similar between the paired tumor and nontumor tissues, though tumor tissues had lower bacterial diversity. *Lactobacillales* was enriched where *Faecalibacterium* was reduced in tumor tissue. In the mucosa-adherent microbiota, *Bifidobacterium, Faecalibacterium,* and *Blautia* were reduced in patients with CRC, whereas *Fusobacterium, Porphyromonas, Peptostreptococcus,* and *Mogibacterium* were enriched. | Chen et al,[56] 2012 |

*(continued on next page)*

**Table 1**
*(continued)*

| Patients | Sample Site | Changes in Microbiota | Study (Author, Year, Reference No.) |
|---|---|---|---|
| 29 Patients with adenoma, 31 patients with CRC, 34 with symptoms but normal colonoscopy, and 31 asymptomatic controls | Colonic biopsies including paired biopsies from tumor and adjacent nontumor tissue in patients with CRC | When assessing for *Escherichia coli* and *E coli*-like bacteria, there was increased presence of intracellular *E coli* in patients with adenoma and CRC. | Swidsinski et al,[53] 1998 |
| 60 Patients with CRC and 119 controls | Fecal samples and colon/rectal biopsies from a subset of 22 patients with CRC and 22 controls | Pyrosequencing on 6 CRC and 6 control samples indicated microbiota differences in patients with CRC vs controls. Higher levels of *Bacteroides/Prevotella* were detected in patients with CRC determined by quantitative PCR. | Sobhani et al,[54] 2011 |
| 104 Patients with CRC | Paired biopsies from tumor and adjacent nontumor tissue in the surgical resection specimen | Whole-genome sequences from 9 tumor/normal pairs revealed that *Fusobacterium* sequences were enriched CRC. Quantitative PCR and 16S rDNA sequence analysis of the remaining 95 CRC/normal tissue pairs confirmed the increased *Fusobacterium*, whereas Bacteroidetes and Firmicutes were depleted in tumors. | Kostic et al,[55] 2012 |
| 99 Patients with CRC | Paired biopsies from tumor and adjacent nontumor tissue in the surgical resection specimen | There was increased *Fusobacterium* in tumor tissues. | Castellarin et al,[57] 2012 |
| 10 Patients with CRC and 11 controls | Fecal samples | There was no significant differences in microbial community structure or diversity between patients with CRC and controls. However, *Bacteroides* and *Prevotella* were relatively underrepresented, whereas there were higher percentages of *Akkermansia muciniphila* in patients with CRC. | Weir et al,[58] 2013 |

| | | | |
|---|---|---|---|
| 344 patients with advanced adenomas (size >10 mm or villous, tubulovillus, or high-grade dysplasia on pathology) and 344 controls | Fecal samples | There was increased abundance of *Enterococcus* and *Streptococcus* species and decreased prevalence of *Roseburia* and *Clostridium* in the patients with adenoma. | Chen et al,[64] 2013 |
| 33 Patients with adenoma and 38 controls | Rectal biopsies | Increased microbial richness with increased abundance of Firmicutes, Bacteroidetes, and Proteobacteria in patients with adenoma. | Sanapareddy et al,[63] 2012 |
| 30 Patients with adenoma, 30 patients with CRC, and 30 controls | Fecal samples | Microbial dysbiosis and enrichment of pathogenic bacteria were seen in patients with adenoma and CRC compared with controls. In patients with adenoma, there were higher relative abundances of *Blautia, Ruminococcus, Clostridium,* and *Lachnospiraceae* compared with CRC. Patients with CRC had higher relative abundances of *Fusobacterium, Bacteroides, Phascolarctobacterium,* and *Porphyromonas* compared with patients with adenoma. | Zackular et al,[59] 2014 |

*Abbreviation:* PCR, polymerase chain reaction.

Recent studies have attempted to define the link between dietary intake, the gut microbiota, and CRC.[52,64] One study found lower levels of butyrate-producing bacteria and decreased fecal SCFAs in meat-eating African Americans, who are at higher risk for CRC, compared with native Africans.[52] In addition, patients with advanced colorectal adenomas were found to have lower dietary fiber intake patterns and consistently lower SCFA levels versus controls.[64] When categorized by dietary fiber intake, low dietary fiber intake remained associated with a deficiency in butyrate-producing bacteria, which could increase the risk for advanced adenomas.[64]

## ANIMAL MODELS

Animal models of CRC allow for investigation of the potential links between GI microbes and risk for colonic neoplasia; specifically, the ability to study these models both in conventional or GF conditions. One of the most common models used is the APC multiple intestinal neoplasia (Min) murine model of colon carcinogenesis. $APC^{Min/+}$ mice possess a point mutation in the murine homolog of the human APC tumor-suppressor gene resulting in spontaneous adenomas, primarily in the small intestine.[69] GF $APC^{Min/+}$ mice have a reduced overall tumor burden including fewer colon tumors versus conventionally housed controls.[70] Exposure to commensal strains, such as enterotoxigenic *Bacteroides fragilis* and *Citrobacter rodentium*, promotes colon tumor formation in $APC^{Min/+}$ mice, whereas a nontoxigenic strain of *Bacteroides fragilis* does not.[71] Furthermore, mono-association with *Bacteroides vulgatus* reduced colorectal tumorigenesis in $IL\text{-}10^{-/-}$ mice versus conventionally housed controls.[72] Thus, when the host genetic background is identical, exposure to different microbial species can lead to altered risk for colon carcinogenesis. This risk can also be modified by antibiotic exposure in models, such as nucleotide-binding oligomerization domain containing 2 (Nod2)$^{-/-}$ mice. $Nod2^{-/-}$ mice have an altered GI microbiota when compared with wild-type (WT) mice and develop more tumors following azoxymethane/dextran sulfate sodium treatment.[73] Antibiotic exposure or fecal transplants from WT mice can abrogate this phenotype.[73] Additionally, WT mice cohoused with $Nod2^{-/-}$ mice exhibit increased tumorigenesis versus separately housed controls.[73] Collectively, these findings suggest that microbial manipulation could be used to abrogate CRC risk if the specific exposures driving the risk are identified.

## SUMMARY

Many factors contribute to the development of GI cancers. Multiple inherited and acquired mutations in epithelial cells have been identified; alterations in risk have also been attributed to environmental exposures, such as diet and now the microbiota. However, identifying whether specific microbes within the complex microbiota are driving the progression to cancer is challenging because of the multidimensional nature of the community, which can be altered by diet and antibiotics and influenced by the genotype of the individual.

Ongoing analyses of the GI microbiota have found patterns that associate with both malignant and premalignant lesions, such as atrophic gastritis and colonic polyps. However, whether these alterations play a direct role in disease development or progression or whether they are markers of underlying epithelial or immune cell dysregulation have yet to be determined. The GI microbiome harbors significant metabolic activity, which can alter dietary nutrients with both beneficial and potentially harmful sequelae. It is tempting to speculate that, in the future, we may identify groups of bacterial taxa that can predict GI disease risk or outcome. These biomarkers could potentially be used to stratify patients towards particular therapeutic regimens, providing further options for using the GI microbiome in the treatment and potentially prevention of GI tract malignancies.

## REFERENCES

1. Blaser MJ. The microbiome revolution. J Clin Invest 2014;124(10):4162–5.
2. Cho I, Blaser MJ. The human microbiome: at the interface of health and disease. Nat Rev Genet 2012;13(4):260–70.
3. Siegel RL, Miller KD, Jemal A. Cancer statistics, 2015. CA Cancer J Clin 2015; 65(1):5–29.
4. de Martel C, Ferlay J, Franceschi S, et al. Global burden of cancers attributable to infections in 2008: a review and synthetic analysis. Lancet Oncol 2012;13(6): 607–15.
5. Plottel CS, Blaser MJ. Microbiome and malignancy. Cell Host Microbe 2011; 10(4):324–35.
6. Ferlay J, Soerjomataram I, Dikshit R, et al. Cancer incidence and mortality worldwide: sources, methods and major patterns in GLOBOCAN 2012. Int J Cancer 2015;136(5):E359–86.
7. Fuchs CS, Mayer RJ. Gastric carcinoma. N Engl J Med 1995;333(1):32–41.
8. Howson CP, Hiyama T, Wynder EL. The decline in gastric cancer: epidemiology of an unplanned triumph. Epidemiol Rev 1986;8:1–27.
9. Blot WJ, Devesa SS, Kneller RW, et al. Rising incidence of adenocarcinoma of the esophagus and gastric cardia. JAMA 1991;265(10):1287–9.
10. Pera M, Cameron AJ, Trastek VF, et al. Increasing incidence of adenocarcinoma of the esophagus and esophagogastric junction. Gastroenterology 1993;104(2): 510–3.
11. Plummer M, Franceschi S, Vignat J, et al. Global burden of gastric cancer attributable to *Helicobacter pylori*. Int J Cancer 2015;136(2):487–90.
12. Wroblewski LE, Peek RM Jr, Wilson KT. *Helicobacter pylori* and gastric cancer: factors that modulate disease risk. Clin Microbiol Rev 2010;23(4):713–39.
13. Linz B, Balloux F, Moodley Y, et al. An African origin for the intimate association between humans and *Helicobacter pylori*. Nature 2007;445(7130):915–8.
14. Amieva M, Peek RM Jr. Pathobiology of *Helicobacter pylori*-induced gastric cancer. Gastroenterology 2016;150(1):64–78.
15. Wroblewski LE, Peek RM Jr. *Helicobacter pylori* in gastric carcinogenesis: mechanisms. Gastroenterol Clin North Am 2013;42(2):285–98.
16. Cover TL, Blanke SR. *Helicobacter pylori* VacA, a paradigm for toxin multifunctionality. Nat Rev Microbiol 2005;3(4):320–32.
17. Boquet P, Ricci V. Intoxication strategy of *Helicobacter pylori* VacA toxin. Trends Microbiol 2012;20(4):165–74.
18. Atherton JC, Cao P, Peek RM Jr, et al. Mosaicism in vacuolating cytotoxin alleles of *Helicobacter pylori*. Association of specific vacA types with cytotoxin production and peptic ulceration. J Biol Chem 1995;270(30):17771–7.
19. Atherton JC, Peek RM Jr, Tham KT, et al. Clinical and pathological importance of heterogeneity in vacA, the vacuolating cytotoxin gene of *Helicobacter pylori*. Gastroenterology 1997;112(1):92–9.
20. Miehlke S, Kirsch C, Agha-Amiri K, et al. The *Helicobacter pylori* vacA s1, m1 genotype and cagA is associated with gastric carcinoma in Germany. Int J Cancer 2000;87(3):322–7.

21. Ma JL, Zhang L, Brown LM, et al. Fifteen-year effects of *Helicobacter pylori*, garlic, and vitamin treatments on gastric cancer incidence and mortality. J Natl Cancer Inst 2012;104(6):488–92.

22. Sheh A, Fox JG. The role of the gastrointestinal microbiome in *Helicobacter pylori* pathogenesis. Gut Microbes 2013;4(6):505–31.

23. Abreu MT, Peek RM Jr. Gastrointestinal malignancy and the microbiome. Gastroenterology 2014;146(6):1534–46.

24. Bik EM, Eckburg PB, Gill SR, et al. Molecular analysis of the bacterial microbiota in the human stomach. Proc Natl Acad Sci U S A 2006;103(3):732–7.

25. Andersson AF, Lindberg M, Jakobsson H, et al. Comparative analysis of human gut microbiota by barcoded pyrosequencing. PLoS One 2008;3(7):e2836.

26. Maldonado-Contreras A, Goldfarb KC, Godoy-Vitorino F, et al. Structure of the human gastric bacterial community in relation to *Helicobacter pylori* status. ISME J 2011;5(4):574–9.

27. Correa P. Human gastric carcinogenesis: a multistep and multifactorial process–first American Cancer Society award lecture on cancer epidemiology and prevention. Cancer Res 1992;52(24):6735–40.

28. Jackson MA, Goodrich JK, Maxan ME, et al. Proton pump inhibitors alter the composition of the gut microbiota. Gut 2015. http://dx.doi.org/10.1136/gutjnl-2015-310861.

29. Imhann F, Bonder MJ, Vich Vila A, et al. Proton pump inhibitors affect the gut microbiome. Gut 2015. http://dx.doi.org/10.1136/gutjnl-2015-310376.

30. Dicksved J, Lindberg M, Rosenquist M, et al. Molecular characterization of the stomach microbiota in patients with gastric cancer and in controls. J Med Microbiol 2009;58(Pt 4):509–16.

31. Eun CS, Kim BK, Han DS, et al. Differences in gastric mucosal microbiota profiling in patients with chronic gastritis, intestinal metaplasia, and gastric cancer using pyrosequencing methods. Helicobacter 2014;19(6):407–16.

32. Yang I, Woltemate S, Piazuelo MB, et al. Different gastric microbiota compositions in two human populations with high and low gastric cancer risk in Colombia. Sci Rep 2016;6:18594.

33. Rolig AS, Cech C, Ahler E, et al. The degree of *Helicobacter pylori*-triggered inflammation is manipulated by preinfection host microbiota. Infect Immun 2013;81(5):1382–9.

34. Sigal M, Rothenberg ME, Logan CY, et al. *Helicobacter pylori* activates and expands Lgr5(+) stem cells through direct colonization of the gastric glands. Gastroenterology 2015;148(7):1392–404.

35. Aebischer T, Fischer A, Walduck A, et al. Vaccination prevents *Helicobacter pylori*-induced alterations of the gastric flora in mice. FEMS Immunol Med Microbiol 2006;46(2):221–9.

36. Tan MP, Kaparakis M, Galic M, et al. Chronic *Helicobacter pylori* infection does not significantly alter the microbiota of the murine stomach. Appl Environ Microbiol 2007;73(3):1010–3.

37. Lofgren JL, Whary MT, Ge Z, et al. Lack of commensal flora in *Helicobacter pylori*-infected INS-GAS mice reduces gastritis and delays intraepithelial neoplasia. Gastroenterology 2011;140(1):210–20.

38. Thomson MJ, Pritchard DM, Boxall SA, et al. Gastric *Helicobacter* infection induces iron deficiency in the INS-GAS mouse. PLoS One 2012;7(11):e50194.

39. Wang J, Fan X, Lindholm C, et al. *Helicobacter pylori* modulates lymphoepithelial cell interactions leading to epithelial cell damage through Fas/Fas ligand interactions. Infect Immun 2000;68(7):4303–11.

40. Lertpiriyapong K, Whary MT, Muthupalani S, et al. Gastric colonisation with a restricted commensal microbiota replicates the promotion of neoplastic lesions by diverse intestinal microbiota in the *Helicobacter pylori* INS-GAS mouse model of gastric carcinogenesis. Gut 2014;63(1):54–63.

41. Peek RM Jr, Blaser MJ. *Helicobacter pylori* and gastrointestinal tract adenocarcinomas. Nat Rev Cancer 2002;2(1):28–37.

42. Yang L, Lu X, Nossa CW, et al. Inflammation and intestinal metaplasia of the distal esophagus are associated with alterations in the microbiome. Gastroenterology 2009;137(2):588–97.

43. Blackett KL, Siddhi SS, Cleary S, et al. Oesophageal bacterial biofilm changes in gastro-oesophageal reflux disease, Barrett's and oesophageal carcinoma: association or causality? Aliment Pharmacol Ther 2013;37(11):1084–92.

44. Bogaert J, Prenen H. Molecular genetics of colorectal cancer. Ann Gastroenterol 2014;27(1):9–14.

45. Vogelstein B, Kinzler KW. The multistep nature of cancer. Trends Genet 1993;9(4):138–41.

46. Dejea C, Wick E, Sears CL. Bacterial oncogenesis in the colon. Future Microbiol 2013;8(4):445–60.

47. Slattery ML, Curtin K, Sweeney C, et al. Diet and lifestyle factor associations with CpG island methylator phenotype and BRAF mutations in colon cancer. Int J Cancer 2007;120(3):656–63.

48. Gill SR, Pop M, Deboy RT, et al. Metagenomic analysis of the human distal gut microbiome. Science 2006;312(5778):1355–9.

49. Marchesi JR, Adams DH, Fava F, et al. The gut microbiota and host health: a new clinical frontier. Gut 2016;65(2):330–9.

50. Keku TO, Dulal S, Deveaux A, et al. The gastrointestinal microbiota and colorectal cancer. Am J Physiol Gastrointest Liver Physiol 2015;308(5):G351–63.

51. Arthur JC, Perez-Chanona E, Muhlbauer M, et al. Intestinal inflammation targets cancer-inducing activity of the microbiota. Science 2012;338(6103):120–3.

52. Ou J, Carbonero F, Zoetendal EG, et al. Diet, microbiota, and microbial metabolites in colon cancer risk in rural Africans and African Americans. Am J Clin Nutr 2013;98(1):111–20.

53. Swidsinski A, Khilkin M, Kerjaschki D, et al. Association between intraepithelial *Escherichia coli* and colorectal cancer. Gastroenterology 1998;115(2):281–6.

54. Sobhani I, Tap J, Roudot-Thoraval F, et al. Microbial dysbiosis in colorectal cancer (CRC) patients. PLoS One 2011;6(1):e16393.

55. Kostic AD, Gevers D, Pedamallu CS, et al. Genomic analysis identifies association of Fusobacterium with colorectal carcinoma. Genome Res 2012;22(2):292–8.

56. Chen W, Liu F, Ling Z, et al. Human intestinal lumen and mucosa-associated microbiota in patients with colorectal cancer. PLoS One 2012;7(6):e39743.

57. Castellarin M, Warren RL, Freeman JD, et al. *Fusobacterium nucleatum* infection is prevalent in human colorectal carcinoma. Genome Res 2012;22(2):299–306.

58. Weir TL, Manter DK, Sheflin AM, et al. Stool microbiome and metabolome differences between colorectal cancer patients and healthy adults. PLoS One 2013;8(8):e70803.

59. Zackular JP, Rogers MA, Ruffin MT, et al. The human gut microbiome as a screening tool for colorectal cancer. Cancer Prev Res 2014;7(11):1112–21.

60. Scanlan PD, Shanahan F, Clune Y, et al. Culture-independent analysis of the gut microbiota in colorectal cancer and polyposis. Environ Microbiol 2008;10(3):789–98.

61. Shen XJ, Rawls JF, Randall T, et al. Molecular characterization of mucosal adherent bacteria and associations with colorectal adenomas. Gut Microbes 2010;1(3):138–47.

62. Marchesi JR, Dutilh BE, Hall N, et al. Towards the human colorectal cancer microbiome. PLoS One 2011;6(5):e20447.

63. Sanapareddy N, Legge RM, Jovov B, et al. Increased rectal microbial richness is associated with the presence of colorectal adenomas in humans. ISME J 2012; 6(10):1858–68.

64. Chen HM, Yu YN, Wang JL, et al. Decreased dietary fiber intake and structural alteration of gut microbiota in patients with advanced colorectal adenoma. Am J Clin Nutr 2013;97(5):1044–52.

65. Greer JB, O'Keefe SJ. Microbial induction of immunity, inflammation, and cancer. Front Physiol 2011;1:168.

66. Vargas AJ, Thompson PA. Diet and nutrient factors in colorectal cancer risk. Nutr Clin Pract 2012;27(5):613–23.

67. Chang PV, Hao L, Offermanns S, et al. The microbial metabolite butyrate regulates intestinal macrophage function via histone deacetylase inhibition. Proc Natl Acad Sci U S A 2014;111(6):2247–52.

68. Louis P, Hold GL, Flint HJ. The gut microbiota, bacterial metabolites and colorectal cancer. Nat Rev Microbiol 2014;12(10):661–72.

69. Moser AR, Pitot HC, Dove WF. A dominant mutation that predisposes to multiple intestinal neoplasia in the mouse. Science 1990;247(4940):322–4.

70. Li Y, Kundu P, Seow SW, et al. Gut microbiota accelerate tumor growth via c-jun and STAT3 phosphorylation in APCMin/+ mice. Carcinogenesis 2012;33(6): 1231–8.

71. Sussman DA, Santaolalla R, Strobel S, et al. Cancer in inflammatory bowel disease: lessons from animal models. Curr Opin Gastroenterol 2012;28(4):327–33.

72. Uronis JM, Muhlbauer M, Herfarth HH, et al. Modulation of the intestinal microbiota alters colitis-associated colorectal cancer susceptibility. PLoS One 2009; 4(6):e6026.

73. Couturier-Maillard A, Secher T, Rehman A, et al. NOD2-mediated dysbiosis predisposes mice to transmissible colitis and colorectal cancer. J Clin Invest 2013; 123(2):700–11.

# Index

*Note:* Page numbers of article titles are in **boldface** type.

## A

Abdominal pain, in NETs, 489
Achalasia, esophageal cancer in, 400
Adenocarcinoma
    esophageal, 400–405
    gastric, **413–428,** 544–547
    pancreatic ductal, **429–445**
    small bowel, **447–457**
Adenoma(s), detection of, colonoscopy for, 464–467
Adenoma detection rate, in CRC, 465–466
Adenomatous polyposis coli, 448–449
Adipokines, in esophageal cancer, 401
Afibercept, for CRC, 469
Alcohol use
    esophageal cancer in, 400–401
    gastric cancer in, 416
Alpha-antitrypsin antigen, 531
American Society for Gastrointestinal Endoscopy, 420
Amsterdam criteria, 512, 519
*APC* gene, 516
    cancer risk of, 510
    in CRC, 460, 547, 552
    in SBA, 448–449
Atrophic gastritis, in *Helicobacter pylori* infections, 419
*ATRXX* gene, 489

## B

BALLAD study, 452
*BAMPR* genes, 510
Bannayan-Riley-Ruvalcaba syndrome, 461
Barrett's esophagus, 401–403, 406, 532–534
Bevacizumab, for CRC, 469
Biomarkers, for NETs, 492–494
Biopsy
    for esophageal cancer, 406
    for PDA, 435
Bleeding, in CRC, 466–467
Blood, for molecular analysis, 535, 537
*BMP3* gene, in CRC, 536
*BMPR1* gene, 461, 517
Boston Bowel Preparation Scale, 467

Gastroenterol Clin N Am 45 (2016) 557–569
http://dx.doi.org/10.1016/S0889-8553(16)30054-1
0889-8553/16/$ – see front matter

Printed and bound by CPI Group (UK) Ltd, Croydon, CR0 4YY

03/10/2024

01040392-0017